THE
BIG BOOK
OF
INFECTIOUS
DISEASE
TRIVIA

THE
BIG BOOK
OF
INFECTIOUS
DISEASE
TRIVIA

Everything You Ever
Wanted to Know about
the World's Worst Pandemics,
Epidemics, and Diseases

KRISTINA WRIGHT

Published in the US by:
ULYSSES PRESS
PO Box 3440
Berkeley, CA 94703
www.ulyssespress.com

ISBN: 978-1-64604-138-1
Library of Congress Control Number: 2020946842

Printed in the United States by Kingery Printing Company
10 9 8 7 6 5 4 3 2 1

Acquisitions editor: Claire Sielaff
Managing editor: Claire Chun
Editor: Kathy Kaiser
Proofreader: Renee Rutledge
Front cover design: Rebecca Lown
Artwork: © nobeastsofierce/shutterstock.com
Interior design: what!design @ whatweb.com

CONTENTS

INTRODUCTION **1**

CHAPTER 1
**UNDERSTANDING INFECTIOUS
DISEASES** **3**

What are infectious diseases? 4

What was the first documented infectious disease? 5

What is the difference between an infectious disease
and a contagious disease? 5

What is botulism, and is it contagious? 7

What is the plague? 8

Has the United States ever had plague? 10

Why isn't plague a big global problem now? Where did it go? 11

What is R0? 12

What is Rt? 13

What is germ theory? 14

How does a disease make the jump from animals to humans? 15

Which zoonotic diseases are most common today? 16

How many human coronaviruses are there? 17

How is rabies transmitted, and which animals transmit the virus? 18

What is herd immunity, and why is it important? .19

What is an asymptomatic carrier? 19

What is the difference between isolation, quarantine, and
social distancing? 20

What is a vaccine, and how does it work? 21

How long have vaccines been around? 21

Is there a vaccine for the plague? 23

How long does it take to develop a vaccine? 24

What was the first disease to be declared eradicated worldwide? 25

Why can't we eradicate all infectious diseases, as we did with
smallpox? 26

If vaccines are so effective, why do outbreaks of vaccine-
preventable diseases still occur? 27

What are the most common vaccine-preventable adult diseases? . . . 28

What are antibiotics, and how do they work? 29

Are antibiotics an effective treatment for infectious diseases? 30

What are antiviral drugs, and how are they used to treat
infectious diseases? 30

What does an allergy to eggs have to do with whether
you can receive certain vaccines? 31

Which infectious diseases were much more common before
vaccines were developed for them? 32

Does every infectious disease have a vaccine? 33

Why are some vaccines more effective than others? And what are
booster shots? 34

Where did whooping cough get its name? 35

How do you know when you have an infectious disease?
Do all infectious diseases have similar symptoms? 36

CHAPTER 2
OUTBREAKS, EPIDEMICS, AND PANDEMICS 39

What does "level of disease" mean? 40

What's the difference between an epidemic and a pandemic? 40

How is a cluster different from an outbreak? 41

What causes an epidemic? 42

What is a zoonotic disease? 43

How is global warming affecting the spread of
infectious diseases? 45

What is a zombie pathogen? 46

Are infectious diseases the top cause of death in the world? 47

What is public health surveillance, and why do we track
the number of deaths caused by infectious diseases? 47

What have been the deadliest pandemics in human history? 48

Could a pandemic on the scale of the Black Death
ever happen again? 50

What are the phases of a pandemic? 50

How do experts determine when a pandemic is over?
What is the difference between a medical end and a
social end to a pandemic? 53

What are biological weapons, and how are they used? 54

Have biological weapons ever been used? 56

What is the Biological Weapons Convention? 57

What was the earliest use of biological warfare? 58

Which country was the first to use biological and chemical
weapons of mass destruction in the modern era?..................... 59

Who was Shirō Ishii, and what was his role in the development of
biological weapons?.. .61

Why do samples of smallpox still exist—and will they ever be
destroyed? 63

CHAPTER 3
EARLY HISTORY OF INFECTIOUS
DISEASES 65

Who was the first person to recognize that infectious diseases
can be transmitted from person to person? 66

Who was Galen, and what is miasma theory? .... .67

What does the Bible say about plague and pestilence? 68

Who were plague doctors—and why did they wear a costume?....... .71

When was quarantining sick people first recognized as a way
to halt the spread of disease? .... .72

Was "Typhoid Mary" a real person? .... .73

What were the three great plague pandemics?...................... 74

Which infectious disease do historians believe killed Alexander the
Great? .... .76

Which infectious diseases did George Washington survive? .... .77

Why and how were Native American populations in the
United States affected by infectious diseases from Europe? 78

How was Fiji devastated by the introduction of measles?............. 80

Why is tuberculosis called the romantic disease?...................... .81

What were tuberculosis sanatoriums, and do they still exist?......... 84

CHAPTER 4
INFECTIOUS DISEASES IN
THE ERA OF MODERN MEDICINE 85

When did our current understanding of infectious diseases begin?.... 86

What infectious disease was rumored to be caused by candy? 87

When were medical face masks first used—and why?................ 88

Why is leprosy also called Hansen's disease? 90

What is PPE? .... .91

What are the different types of face masks, and how can
they protect me from becoming infected with COVID-19?............ 92

What does MMR stand for in the MMR vaccine? 93

What is the 80/20 rule? 93

What is a super spreader?.. 94

What vaccines do we have now to protect us from the diseases our grandparents may have experienced when they were kids? 95

What is the difference between a bacterial infection and a viral infection? 97

What is the CDC—and what do they do? 99

How does the World Health Organization look out for the global population? 100

What is the National Institutes of Health? 101

What is the Food and Drug Administration? 101

What is the difference between eradicating a disease and eliminating a disease? 102

What is mad cow disease? Can a person get it by eating beef?...... 104

What's the difference between chicken pox and shingles? And if you've had chicken pox, are you more likely to get shingles? 105

CHAPTER 5
EVERYTHING WE KNOW ABOUT INFLUENZA *107*

Why was the strain of influenza that caused the 1918 pandemic called the Spanish flu?.. 108

Did scientists reconstruct the virus that caused the 1918 influenza pandemic?.. 109

How did the 1918 influenza pandemic affect life expectancy? 109

When was the first flu vaccine created?...............................110

How many different types of influenza virus are there?...............111

How are different influenza viruses named? 112

Who should get a flu vaccine, and how many people get the vaccine each year? 113

Why does the flu vaccine have to be redesigned every year? 114

Which flu viruses have caused pandemics? 115

Can you get the flu from the flu shot?...............................117

Is the stomach flu really the flu?......................................118

How serious is the flu in any given year? How many people die of the flu each year? 120

What is the difference between the flu and the common cold?.......121

Why is there a "flu season," and does that mean you can't catch the flu at other times of the year? 122

CHAPTER 6

SEXUALLY TRANSMITTED DISEASES AND THE HIV/AIDS EPIDEMIC 125

What's the difference between an STI (sexually transmitted infection) and an STD (sexually transmitted disease)?............. 126

How common are sexually transmitted infections? 127

What is the difference between HIV and AIDS?..................... 129

When and where do scientists think HIV likely originated? 129

Where were the first cases of HIV/AIDS identified in the United States? 130

How did HIV and AIDS get their names, and when was HIV first identified as the virus that causes AIDS? 131

How has HIV/AIDS been portrayed in the media and pop culture?.... 132

Is there a cure for HIV? Will there ever be a cure?.................... 134

Will there ever be an HIV vaccine? 135

Is HIV/AIDS still a global health concern? 136

CHAPTER 7

INFECTIOUS DISEASES AROUND THE WORLD. 139

What are tropical diseases, and why do they occur in warmer parts of the world?... 140

What are diseases of poverty and neglected tropical diseases? 140

How has the advent of air travel affected the spread of infectious diseases? 142

What is Ebola virus, and where does it get its name?............... 143

Have there been any cases of Ebola virus disease in the United States? 146

Why is it called yellow fever?..................................... 146

What does gin and tonic have to do with preventing malaria?.......147

Which insects transmit diseases, and what diseases do they transmit? 148

How did King Tut die? 149

CHAPTER 8

LIVING HISTORY 151

When will the COVID-19 pandemic end?........................... 152

How did COVID-19 create a coin shortage?........................ 152

Did scientists predict the COVID-19 pandemic? Why weren't we ready? 153

What is meant by the term *novel coronavirus*? 154

Why is it called COVID-19? Why do the virus and the disease have
different names? 154

How did COVID-19 start? 155

What's the difference between the virus that causes COVID-19 and
previously identified coronaviruses? 155

What are the similarities and differences between the novel
coronavirus and influenza viruses? 156

What is the test for COVID-19? 159

What are comorbidities? 160

What is contact tracing? 160

How can technology be used to manage contact tracing? 161

Can we use the pandemic flu of 1918 as a model for what to
expect from COVID-19? 162

How long will it take for a COVID-19 vaccine to become available? . . 163

What is Operation Warp Speed? 164

Why was COVID-19 called the Wuhan virus and the Chinese
virus before it was called COVID-19? 165

CHAPTER 9

INFECTIOUS DISEASES AND PANDEMICS IN POP CULTURE *167*

Who is Anthony Fauci, MD? 168

Is there really a horror movie about the COVID-19 pandemic? 169

Does the song "A Spoonful of Sugar" in *Mary Poppins* reference a
particular disease? 170

Why were blood tests once required before a marriage license
could be issued? 171

Is flesh-eating bacteria a real thing? 172

Why does the World Health Organization (WHO) have global
public health days? 174

What trends has the COVID-19 pandemic inspired? Why? 174

What do Christmas Seals have to do with tuberculosis? 175

Was Bram Stoker's *Dracula* based on an infectious disease? 176

What is the "miracle toxin?" 178

What novels and movies feature plotlines about infectious
diseases and pandemics? 178

Why does the CDC have a zombie preparedness plan?
Could a zombie apocalypse really happen? 180

Who were the first public figures to test positive for COVID-19?
Have any famous people died of COVID-19? 181

CHAPTER 10
HOW TO STAY HEALTHY **185**

What song should you sing to make sure you have thoroughly washed your hands? 186

Are there any home remedies that actually work to prevent a cold or the flu? 186

What is the difference between raw milk and milk that has been pasteurized? 187

Does chicken soup cure the common cold? And does it matter whether it's Grandma's homemade soup or store-bought? 188

What does "Feed a cold, starve a fever" mean—and does it work? . . . 189

Do bedbugs transmit infectious diseases? 190

What is the best way to protect yourself against an infectious disease? 190

Is it true that "Ring around the Rosie" was about the Black Death? 191

Why do some countries require pets from foreign countries be quarantined upon entry? 192

What is tetanus, and why are we always being told to get a tetanus shot? 193

How does deforestation contribute to the increase of infectious diseases? 195

Can you catch an infectious disease from touching a surface (such as in a public restroom) that has been contaminated by a virus? 196

BIBLIOGRAPHY AND FURTHER READING **197**

ACKNOWLEDGMENTS **225**

ABOUT THE AUTHOR **227**

INTRODUCTION

WHY ARE WE TALKING ABOUT INFECTIOUS DISEASES?

Welcome to the world of infectious diseases! You'll want to wash your hands and put on a face mask before you dive into this germ pool.

Infectious diseases have plagued humankind since the dawn of time. From the ubiquity of the common cold to malaria, dengue fever, and other diseases that spread like wildfire in tropical climates, communities have endured a dizzying variety of person-to-person and animal-to-person diseases.

Although some infectious diseases are no more than an inconvenience to be weathered with a combination of rest, fluids, over-the-counter medications, and a subscription to Netflix, other diseases have caused—and continue to cause—widespread illness and death, with no cure in sight.

The Big Book of Infectious Disease Trivia is filled with information about the history of infectious diseases and how they have affected populations around the globe.

These diseases have not only influenced how people live, work, and travel, but have also led to the development of cutting-edge science and the creation of medical disciplines, such as epidemiology and virology.

From the familiar diseases, such as influenza, to the ancient diseases, such as leprosy, to the oddly named diseases, such as mad cow disease, to the disease caused by a novel (new) coronavirus, COVID-19, *The Big Book of Infectious Disease Trivia* digs into the mind-blowing facts and obscure details about many infectious diseases, past and present, while offering insight into what our future holds.

As we move into a new normal with COVID-19 and face a future in which words such as *social distancing* and *self-quarantine* will certainly linger in our collective consciousness, it's important to remember that our ancestors were here before and, even in times of great uncertainty, we can be guided by their fortitude and wisdom. (And comforted by Grandma's recipe for chicken noodle soup.)

For anyone who has ever uttered the words "I feel like I have the plague" or wondered how COVID-19 is really different from seasonal influenza, *The Big Book of Infectious Disease Trivia* will answer all of your questions about infectious diseases, as well as covering the strange and bizarre questions you may never have thought to ask.

On this bumpy ride through history, hand sanitizer is a necessity and Anthony Fauci, MD, is our best friend. Are you ready? Good, face masks on, and let's go!

CHAPTER 1

UNDERSTANDING INFECTIOUS DISEASES

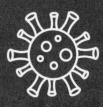

A Layperson's Guide to Disease Terminology and the Basics of Epidemiology

Question: What are infectious diseases?

Answer: Infectious diseases are disorders caused by organisms, such as bacteria, fungi, parasites, or viruses. Infectious diseases can be transmitted in a variety of ways: Some can be passed from person to person, while others are transmitted by insects or animals. Still others can be transmitted through the consumption of contaminated food or water, or even through exposure to certain organisms in the environment.

Many infectious diseases, such as chicken pox, measles, tuberculosis, and pertussis (whooping cough), can be prevented by vaccines administered starting in childhood. Frequent and thorough handwashing can also prevent people from catching or transmitting many infectious diseases. In fact, handwashing alone can reduce the risk of catching a respiratory illness, such as influenza or the common cold, by as much as 45 percent.

Many infectious diseases present as mild infections and will often respond to a combination of rest, fluids, and over-the-counter medications. Some infections, however, can become life-threatening and may require hospitalization.

Signs and symptoms of an infectious disease can vary depending on the organism that has caused the infection, but the most frequent symptoms seen in many infectious diseases include fever and fatigue.

Question: What was the first documented infectious disease?

Answer: As long as there have been people, there have been infectious diseases. Leprosy was first recorded in India around 600 BCE, but molecular evidence suggests the disease may have originated in Africa as far back as the Paleolithic period (2.5 million years ago to 10,000 years ago).

Caused by the bacteria *Mycobacteria leprae*, or *M. leprae*, leprosy still exists in the modern era, but it is not highly contagious. Children are more likely than adults to get leprosy, with the infection being transmitted through repeated contact with droplets from the nose and mouth of someone with untreated leprosy.

According to the World Health Organization (WHO), there are currently only around 180,000 cases of leprosy worldwide, mostly in Africa and Asia. In the United States, around one hundred people are diagnosed with leprosy each year, most of them in California, Hawaii, the South, and some US territories.

Question: What is the difference between an infectious disease and a contagious disease?

Answer: *Infectious* and *contagious* are often used interchangeably when referring to disease transmission, but the two words actually have different meanings. All contagious diseases are infectious, but not all infectious diseases are contagious.

Infectious diseases are illnesses caused by microscopic germs, such as bacteria, fungi, or viruses, that enter the body and cause an infection. Some infectious diseases are spread by contact with an infected person or animal, or by contact with their bodily fluids. Still other infectious diseases can be spread by contact with a contaminated object, such as a tissue, water fountain, or door handle; by contact with contaminated food, water, air, or soil; or by contact with disease-carrying insects or animals.

Infectious diseases that are easily spread through person-to-person contact are called contagious, or communicable, diseases. These are examples of contagious infectious diseases:

- Chicken pox
- Coronavirus
- Ebola
- Hantavirus
- Hepatitis A and B
- Human immunodeficiency virus/acquired immunodeficiency syndrome (HIV/AIDS)
- Influenza
- Measles
- Methicillin-resistant *Staphylococcus aureus* (MRSA)
- Pertussis (whooping cough)
- Pneumonia
- Smallpox
- Sexually transmitted diseases (STDs)
- Tuberculosis
- West Nile virus
- Zika

Noncontagious infectious diseases include some that are transmitted by insects or that are foodborne or waterborne. Lyme disease, for example, is transmitted through the bite of an infected tick but cannot be passed from person to person.

Similarly, dengue fever is a virus that is caused by a mosquito biting a person infected with the disease and then transmitting the disease by biting other people. Dengue fever cannot be transmitted from person to person.

Question: What is botulism, and is it contagious?

Answer: Botulism is an infectious disease that is not contagious. Although rare, it is a potentially life-threatening illness caused by neurotoxins made by *Clostridium botulinum*, a common bacterium found in soil and ocean sediment around the world. Usually, the bacteria exist as dormant spores, but under the right conditions, the spores can germinate into active bacteria, multiply, and produce toxins. Botulinum toxin is one of the most poisonous biological substances known.

Fewer than two hundred cases of botulism are reported annually in the United States, with infant botulism accounting for 75 percent of all botulism cases.

There are five main kinds of botulism:

1. Foodborne botulism: This form of botulism is caused by toxins that can be transmitted when people eat contaminated foods. Contamination can occur when food is improperly handled during preparation or storage. For instance, foods with a low acid content are the most frequent source of botulism cases related to home-canned food. Such low-acid foods include asparagus, beets, corn, green beans, and potatoes.

2. Wound botulism: A wound that isn't properly cleaned and cared for can become infected by the toxin that causes botulism. This form of botulism can occur from injecting illicit drugs or after traumatic injuries or surgeries.

3. Infant botulism: The bacteria that causes botulism can be found in the environment, including in dirt and dust (even after cleaning). But most healthy children and adults can safely ingest botulism spores without becoming sick. In some cases, infants can get botulism when the botulism spores move through their digestive tract, growing and producing the botulism toxin. Because infant botulism has been associated with babies ingesting raw honey, the Food and Drug Administration (FDA) advises parents not to give honey to children younger than one year old.

4. Adult intestinal colonization botulism (or adult intestinal toxemia botulism): Extremely rare and believed to be similar to infant botulism, this is a form of botulism that scientists are still working to understand. People who have health conditions that affect the intestines might be at greater risk.

5. Iatrogenic botulism: This type of botulism is caused by an overdose of Botox, a neurotoxic protein used for medical and cosmetic purposes.

Question: What is the plague?

Answer: The term *plague* has been used colloquially to describe everything from divine biblical events to contemporary malaise. But the plague is actually a very real infectious disease that affects humans and other mammals. Caused by the bacterial toxin *Yersinia pestis*, plague is spread from infected rodents—most often rats—to humans through flea bites. Plague can also spread from one person to another through cough droplets from an infected person.

There are three forms of plague:

- Bubonic plague
- Pneumonic plague
- Septicemic plague

The diagnosis of one of the three forms of plague depends on where the infection is found in the body. With bubonic plague, the infection is in the lymph nodes. For pneumonic plague, the infection is in the lungs. And with septicemic plague, the infection is in the blood.

Plague has, well, *plagued* humankind for millennia. In 2018, researchers discovered the oldest known strain of the bacterium *Yersinia pestis* in a five-thousand-year-old tomb in Sweden. Their findings suggest that plague may have been responsible for the first major pandemic in human history, devastating settlements throughout ancient Europe at the end of the Stone Age.

More recently, the Black Plague, also referred to as the Black Death, ravaged Eurasia and North Africa in the fourteenth century. A form of bubonic plague, the Black Plague is estimated to have killed as much as a third of the European population in just four years, from 1347 to 1351.

Despite its ancient origins, the plague still lives on in the modern era. Between one thousand and two thousand cases of plague are reported to the World Health

Organization each year, but the actual number of unreported cases in poorer populations around the world is assumed to be much higher. Although there is currently no vaccine available to prevent the plague, the development of antibiotics has greatly reduced the mortality rate of plague.

Plague is diagnosed through samples of a patient's blood, sputum, or lymph node aspirate. Each form of plague has its own set of symptoms, but general symptoms of plague can include fever, chills, weakness, headaches, body aches, and swollen lymph nodes.

Question: **Has the United States ever had plague?**

Answer: Historically, significantly higher numbers of plague cases have been documented in other parts of the world, most recently in Africa and Asia, but the United States hasn't entirely escaped the reach of the plague. Rat-infested steamships from affected areas of the world first introduced plague into the United States in 1900, causing epidemics to break out in several port cities. Although it's been nearly a century since the most recent urban plague, experienced by Los Angeles in 1924–25, plague still hasn't been entirely eliminated in the United States.

Once urban rats spread plague to rural rodent species, plague cases began popping up in more remote areas of the western United States. An average of seven human plague cases are reported in the United States each year, with a range of one to seventeen cases each year. More than 80 percent of the plague cases diagnosed in the United States are bubonic plague.

Most reported cases of plague occur in the western part of the country, in two specific regions: northern New Mexico, northern Arizona, and southern Colorado; and California, southern Oregon, and far western Nevada. Although plague can occur at any time of the year, most cases reported in the United States are transmitted from late spring to early fall, when people are most likely to be out-doors and exposed to wild rodents, who may be infected.

Question: **Why isn't plague a big global problem now? Where did it go?**

Answer: After two thousand years, three major pandemics, and millions of lives lost, no one really knows what caused the bubonic plague to fade away.

Some scholars hypothesize that cold weather eventually killed off the fleas that transmitted the plague bacterium or that a change in the rats who carried the plague may have limited how the plague was spread. Originally carried by black rats found in urban areas, by the nineteenth century the plague was more likely to be found in brown rats, who are stronger, larger, and more likely to live in rural areas, away from humans. Likewise, communities took measures to prevent plague, such as using housing materials that were inhospitable to rats and implementing quarantines during outbreaks.

Another theory is that the plague bacterium *Yersinia pestis* may have evolved to be a less deadly strain of bacteria. Whatever the reason for the end of the most recent plague pandemic and the reduction in the global number of plague transmissions, the plague has never entirely faded away. Cases of plague are still reported worldwide, with more than three thousand cases reported from 2010 to 2015, including nearly six hundred deaths.

The three countries where plague is most endemic are the Democratic Republic of the Congo, Madagascar, and Peru.

Question: What is R0?

Answer: R0 is a mathematical term that researchers use to identify how contagious an infectious disease may be. Put another way, it is a measure used to quantify the potential transmission of an epidemic.

Pronounced "R naught" or "R zero," it is the basic reproduction number (also known as the basic reproduction ratio or the basic reproductive rate) of a disease.

An infectious disease reproduces itself when it is transmitted from an infected person to other people. The R0 of a particular infection reflects the expected number of people who will contract the disease from a single person. The R0 of an infection applies to a susceptible population, or people who have neither been infected with a particular disease nor received a vaccination against it.

When it comes to R0, 1 is the magic number. With an R0 of 1, each infected person is expected to transmit the disease to one other person. If a disease has an R0 less than 1, a disease epidemic will eventually fade away on its own. On the other hand, an R0 greater than 1 means the disease could grow exponentially and become a serious public health situation.

A seasonal influenza infection with an R0 of 1.3 would mean that every person with the infection would go on to infect 1.3 people. Or, to use bigger numbers, a 1.3 R0 tells us that 1,000 people infected with an influenza virus will transmit that infection to around 1,300 people. That doesn't seem so bad until you consider that a tenth-generation, thirty-day outbreak of the flu could infect as many as 42,621 people.

An R0 value is not a biological constant—it is an estimation and a starting point for predicting the behavior of a virus in the absence of human and environmental factors. The R0 does not remain static, it changes and fluctuates, particularly at the beginning of an emergence and at the end of an outbreak. An R0 value can be affected by a number of different factors, such as environmental conditions and the behavior of infected populations. In fact, the R0 can even vary between different strains of an infectious disease.

Question: What is Rt?

Answer: While R0 is the basic reproductive number of a virus and represents the average spread of a disease throughout a population, Rt is the time-varying actual (or effective) reproductive number of disease transmission. Rt is used to track the evolution of transmission in real time, allowing researchers to have an accurate and up-to-date record of the infection rate.

By reflecting how a disease is spreading throughout a population in real time, Rt aids the effectiveness of targeted public health policies and community interventions, such as social distancing. As the Rt of a disease epidemic changes, for better or worse, interventions can be lifted or tightened accordingly. Understanding and utilizing Rt is an important part of making public health policies. Individuals in a community can also use the information about Rt shared by public health officials to make personal decisions about planning, traveling to, or attending large events.

Question: What is germ theory?

Answer: The word *germ* refers to any type of microorganism (an organism that can be viewed only under a microscope) that can cause disease. The germ theory of disease is the scientifically accepted principle that infectious diseases are spread via such microorganisms. These microorganisms are known as pathogens, or germs.

The basic tenets of germ theory were first introduced by a variety of physicians in the late Middle Ages. In 1762, Vienna physician Marcus von Plenciz (1705–86) advanced the germ theory of disease by hypothesizing that each known disease was caused by a different organism within the human body. Unfortunately, von Plenciz had no proof to support his forward-thinking hypothesis, and germ theory was widely scorned by the scientists and doctors of his time—most of whom continued to support the idea of disease transmission via "bad air," or Galen's miasma theory (see page 67).

But the germ theory grew with time and research. John Snow, an English physician considered to be a founder of modern epidemiology, was skeptical of Galen's miasma theory as an explanation for the spread of diseases such as cholera and bubonic plague. In 1854 Snow traced an outbreak of cholera in London to a specific water pump in a Soho neighborhood and curbed the spread of the disease by removing the handle of the water pump.

Further research and development of germ theory continued with Louis Pasteur in the late 1850s and Robert Koch in the 1880s. Their work ushered in a golden era of microbiology and, gradually, the miasma theory that had been so widely supported for so long fell out of favor, and germ theory took its place.

Question: **How does a disease make the jump from animals to humans?**

Answer: Diseases that can be passed from animals to humans are called zoonotic diseases. Most of the known infectious diseases are zoonotic diseases and are caused by harmful pathogens, such as bacteria, fungi, parasites, or viruses, which can be spread from animals to humans in a variety of ways, including the following:

Transmission by direct contact: Coming into contact with an infected animal's bodily fluids, including blood, feces, mucus, or urine. Contact can include being bitten or scratched by an infected animal, as well as petting or touching such an animal.

Transmission by indirect contact: Coming into contact with objects or surfaces that have been contaminated with an infected animal's germs. These areas might include plants and soil, as well as pet habitats, such as a barn, chicken coop, or aquarium tank, or the animal's food or water dishes.

Foodborne transmission: Eating or drinking something that has been contaminated with an infected animal's germs. This can include eating undercooked meat or eggs, drinking unpasteurized milk, or eating or drinking something that has been contaminated by feces from an infected animal.

Vector-borne transmission: Being bitten by a disease-carrying insect, such as a flea, mosquito, or tick.

Question: Which zoonotic diseases are most common today?

Answer: There are many zoonotic diseases in the world, but you might not have heard of some of them. The zoonotic diseases of greatest concern in the United States are these:

Zoonotic influenza: Influenza A viruses are found in many types of animals, including cats, chickens, ducks, and horses. It's unusual for people to get influenza infections directly from animals, but some human outbreaks are caused by avian influenza A viruses.

Salmonellosis: Food is the most common source of salmonella bacteria, causing around 1.35 million human infections in the United States every year.

West Nile virus (WNV): This virus is most commonly spread to humans by the bite of an infected mosquito. Not all mosquitoes carry West Nile virus.

Plague: Caused by the bacterium *Yersinia pestis*, plague is transmitted by a flea that once lived on an infected rodent and now carries the bacterium, or by an infected animal.

Rabies: Caused by the rabies virus, rabies is most often transmitted to humans through bites from infected animals.

Brucellosis: Caused by bacteria, brucellosis can be transmitted to humans when they consume undercooked meat or unpasteurized dairy products. It can also be transmitted when humans breathe in the bacteria of or touch the skin or mucous membranes of an infected animal.

Lyme disease: Most often caused by the bacterium *Borrelia burgdorferi* or, more rarely, *Borrelia mayonii*, Lyme disease is transmitted to people through the bite of infected black-legged ticks.

Emerging coronaviruses, including severe acute respiratory syndrome (SARS) and Middle East respiratory syndrome (MERS): Scientists believe that all human coronaviruses (HCoVs) have zoonotic origins, including bats, mice, and domestic animals. A coronavirus can be spread through respiratory droplets, feces that come in contact with the mouth, or infected surfaces.

Question: **How many human coronaviruses are there?**

Scientists have identified seven different types of human coronaviruses (HCoVs). All of these HCoVs have zoonotic origins, most of them bats:

- HCoV-229E
- HCoV-OC43
- SARS-CoV
- HCoV-NL63
- HCoV-HKU1
- MERS-CoV
- SARS-CoV-2 (the virus that causes COVID-19)

Prior to 2003, two human coronaviruses were known to cause mild symptoms and a cold-like illness. Outbreaks of severe acute respiratory syndrome (SARS) and Middle East respiratory syndrome (MERS) have demonstrated the potential for HCoVs to cause serious, life-threatening infections requiring hospitalization.

Question: How is rabies transmitted, and which animals transmit the virus?

Answer: Rabies is a zoonotic viral disease that occurs in more than 150 countries. Although the disease can be prevented with a rabies vaccination, once clinical symptoms have appeared, rabies is almost always fatal.

This virus is spread through direct contact—via broken skin or mucous membranes in the eyes, nose, or mouth—with the saliva, brain tissue, or nervous tissue of an infected animal. The rabies virus infects the mammalian central nervous system, causing disease in the brain that usually leads to death.

The most common way rabies is transmitted to humans is through an animal bite. Any mammal can get rabies, but in the United States, the majority of rabies cases reported to the Centers for Disease Control and Prevention (CDC) each year originate with wild animals, such as bats, foxes, skunks, and raccoons.

Although vaccination has made rabies rare in domestic animals in the United States, dogs account for 99 percent of rabies cases worldwide. Rabies infections are responsible for thousands of human deaths each year, most often in Asia and Africa.

Question: What is herd immunity, and why is it important?

Answer: Herd immunity, which is also called herd protection, happens when a large portion of a population becomes immune to a disease, which then reduces the likelihood that the disease will continue to spread to those who are not immune. The percentage of the community that needs to be immune in order for the entire population to achieve herd immunity varies from disease to disease, but in general, herd immunity requires 70 to 90 percent immunity.

Once herd immunity is established, the entire community has greater protection from the disease.

In some cases, herd immunity can be achieved through vaccination. For instance, administering childhood vaccines for infectious diseases, such as chicken pox, measles, mumps, and polio, have helped establish herd immunity in the United States. Vaccination campaigns encourage people to get recommended vaccines and thus help attain herd immunity in their community, which works to protect vulnerable populations who are unable to be vaccinated or who have delayed vaccination.

Question: What is an asymptomatic carrier?

Answer: A person, animal, or other organism that is infected with a pathogen but does not exhibit any symptoms of sickness is called an asymptomatic carrier (or just a carrier). An asymptomatic carrier may present as healthy while still being able to transmit the pathogen to others. The widespread transmission of common infectious diseases, such as influenza, tuberculosis, and HIV, can be attributed to asymptomatic carriers.

An asymptomatic carrier might never develop symptoms of the disease or might develop them at a slower rate than a person who is symptomatic. Researchers are working to understand the dormancy period of pathogens so that they can mitigate the spread of infectious diseases by asymptomatic carriers.

Question: **What is the difference between isolation, quarantine, and social distancing?**

Answer: The terms *isolation*, *quarantine*, and *social distancing* are often used in reference to slowing the spread of an infectious disease.

- Isolation separates people who are sick with a contagious infectious disease from people who are not sick in order to prevent the spread of the disease.

- Quarantine separates and limits the movement of people who have been (or may have been) exposed to a contagious disease to see if they become sick. A person who is quarantined may be tested to determine whether he or she is an asymptomatic carrier, or this individual may opt to self-quarantine until the incubation period for the disease has passed.

- Social distancing is maintaining space between yourself and people outside your household to prevent the spread of disease. Social distancing may be a matter of maintaining a specific distance (generally six feet) between individuals who do not live in the same household, or it could involve avoiding large gatherings, such as concerts or parties, where many people are in close contact.

Question: **What is a vaccine, and how does it work?**

Answer: A vaccine is developed using the same germs that cause the disease. Vaccines are different from other types of medicines because they're designed to improve immunity and prevent a particular disease rather than curing it. For that reason, vaccines are received before exposure to an infectious disease.

The germs used to develop a vaccine may be either weakened or killed so they do not cause illness, or the vaccine may contain only a small part of the germ that causes the disease. Once administered, a vaccine stimulates the body's immune system to produce antibodies in a way that is similar to—but safer than—the way the immune system is engaged after a disease is contracted. Once you receive a vaccine, you develop an immunity to a particular disease without having to get that disease.

Question: **How long have vaccines been around?**

Answer: Although English physician and scientist Edward Jenner (1749–1823), who created the first smallpox vaccine, is considered the founder of vaccinology, evidence suggests that the foundation for vaccines actually began much earlier. In fact, as early as 1000 CE, the Chinese used smallpox material as a way to offer immunity to the disease. This technique is called variolation and was also practiced in Africa and Turkey before making its way to Great Britain in 1721.

Jenner hit upon the idea of using cowpox material to provide immunity to smallpox after observing that milkmaids who had previously caught cowpox did not catch smallpox. In 1796, he tested his theory by inoculating a boy with cowpox pustule liquid obtained from the hand of a milkmaid. Jenner continued to conduct experiments using cowpox material and, in 1801, published "On the Origin of the Vaccine Inoculation," his work on the development of a smallpox vaccine.

In the 1870s and 1880s, the work of French biologist, microbiologist, and chemist Louis Pasteur (1822–95) and German physician and microbiologist Robert Koch (1843–1910) led to a golden era of microbiology, which lasted into the early 1900s. Due to their substantial contributions to the field of microbiology, Pasteur and Koch are considered the founders of medical bacteriology, even though the two had a legendary rivalry.

By the 1930s, vaccines and antitoxins had been developed for anthrax, cholera, plague, tetanus, tuberculosis, typhoid, and more. Vaccine research and development continued at a rapid pace into the middle of the twentieth century, leading researchers to target common childhood diseases, such as polio, measles, mumps, and rubella.

Question: Is there a vaccine for the plague?

Answer: Vaccines for plague have been developed and used since the late-nineteenth century, but the effectiveness of these vaccines has never been determined. Currently, although an oral vaccine has been shown to be effective against pneumonic—but not bubonic—plague, there is no licensed plague vaccine available. But although it seems unlikely the world will see another plague pandemic, researchers are still diligently working on an effective vaccine.

One reason is that a large plague outbreak occurred in Madagascar in 2017. More than two thousand cases of plague (with more than two hundred deaths) were reported on the island, contributing to the plague being recognized internationally as a reemerging disease.

Another reason for the research into an effective plague vaccine is the potential for the plague to be weaponized. *Yersinia pestis*, the bacterium strain that causes the plague, has already had documented use as a biological weapon and, during the Cold War, the CDC identified aerosolized *Y. pestis* as a bioweapon with a high threat level. For these reasons, researchers continue to work on developing an effective vaccine treatment, which possibly will be a combination of different types of vaccines that support different kinds of immunity.

Question: How long does it take to develop a vaccine?

Answer: Developing a new vaccine is a lengthy and complex process that can take ten to fifteen years and cost as much as $500 million.

Vaccine development and testing in the United States follow a standard set of stages with increasing regulations and oversight as the vaccine gets further along in the process of development.

These are the stages of vaccine development:

1. Exploratory

2. Preclinical

3. Clinical development

   - *Phase I*: The trial vaccine is given to small groups of people

   - *Phase II*: The study is expanded, with the vaccine given to people who share characteristics (such as age) with those for whom the vaccine is intended

   - *Phase III*: The vaccine is given to thousands of people and tested for efficacy and safety

4. Regulatory review and approval

5. Manufacturing and delivery

6. Quality control

Many vaccines undergo a Phase IV after the vaccine is approved and licensed, which includes formal, ongoing studies to determine the safety and effectiveness of the vaccine and monitor reports of its adverse effects.

Question: What was the first disease to be declared eradicated worldwide?

Answer: Over time, Edward Jenner's smallpox vaccine continued to be refined and utilized throughout the world. Sometime in the 1800s, *Vaccinia virus* (a virus that belongs to the poxvirus family) replaced the use of cowpox in the smallpox inoculation. Vaccination eventually replaced variolation as the preferred practice of providing immunity to smallpox.

In 1959, the World Health Organization (WHO) put an initial plan into effect with the goal of eradicating smallpox worldwide. At that point, the disease had already been eliminated in North America and Europe, making it conceivable that the disease could be eliminated in other parts of the world. Unfortunately, a number of stumbling blocks affected the WHO's attempts to rid the rest of the world of smallpox—including a lack of funding, personnel, and commitment from countries, and a shortage of vaccine donations. As a result, smallpox outbreaks continued into the mid-1960s in countries throughout South America, Africa, and Asia.

In 1967 the Intensified Eradication Program was initiated, with a renewed goal of eliminating smallpox worldwide. The increased production of a higher-quality, freeze-dried vaccine, the development of the bifurcated needle, the formulation of a system of detection and investigation of cases, and a widespread vaccination campaign all led to the success of the new eradication program.

It took almost two hundred years from Edward Jenner's first experiments with smallpox vaccination, but the last case of naturally acquired smallpox occurred in Somalia in October 1977. On May 8, 1980, the thirty-third World Health Assembly officially declared the global eradication of smallpox.

Question: Why can't we eradicate all infectious diseases, as we did with smallpox?

Answer: Efforts to eradicate all infectious diseases are ongoing worldwide. But when it comes to eradication, a number of factors must be in place—and it took a perfect storm of favorable circumstances to eradicate smallpox.

For one thing, smallpox is not a zoonotic disease, meaning the virus that causes it, *Variola major*, has no animal host. Eliminating smallpox in humans meant the total elimination of the disease, with no risk of it returning by way of spread among animal populations, which could then transmit it to humans.

Smallpox also presents with a set of unique symptoms, including a rash that develops into pustules, making a smallpox infection easily identifiable. Being able to easily and quickly identify a disease aids in public health measures, such as quarantining and contract tracing.

Finally, the development of an effective vaccine with lifelong protection, coupled with aggressive global vaccination campaigns that had strong financial and community support, were big factors in the eradication of smallpox.

Question: If vaccines are so effective, why do outbreaks of vaccine-preventable diseases still occur?

Answer: As well as eradicating smallpox worldwide, vaccines have greatly reduced the rate of a number of other infectious diseases, both in the United States and around the world. But that doesn't mean a disease that has been controlled by vaccines can't make a comeback. In fact, several countries have seen a sudden and dramatic uptick in certain infectious diseases following a decrease in immunization rates.

In 1974, around 80 percent of Japanese children were inoculated against pertussis (whooping cough). That year, Japan reported only 393 cases of whooping cough and no deaths related to the disease. Within five years, the immunization rate plummeted to just 10 percent. As a result, Japan saw a startling 13,000 cases of whooping cough in 1979, with 41 deaths attributed to the disease. Thankfully, the rate of infection once again dropped when routine vaccinations increased.

The 2019 measles outbreaks throughout the United States are another unfortunate example of a vaccine-preventable disease making an unwanted return. In 2000, after three decades of widespread vaccine use to protect against the highly infectious disease, measles was considered eliminated from the United States.

Predictably, a drop in routine inoculations in the past two decades has led to an increase in the number of reported measles cases. In 2019, measles outbreaks occurred in several US states, including New York, Washington, Michigan, New Jersey, California, Georgia, Maryland, and

Pennsylvania, with additional cases reported in more than thirty other states. The number of cases in New York City led Mayor Bill de Blasio to declare a public health emergency and require unvaccinated residents living in certain zip codes to get the vaccine or face a fine.

These examples point out the benefits of widespread vaccination. Vaccines not only protect the people who have been inoculated against the disease, but also contribute to the herd immunity of the larger community. The more people who are inoculated against a particular infectious disease, the more people who cannot receive vaccines—including the very young, the elderly, and the immunocompromised, as well as those whose vaccines have been delayed—are protected.

Question: What are the most common vaccine-preventable adult diseases?

Answer: Vaccines aren't only for children. Although many vaccines are administered in childhood, adults can also benefit from getting vaccines they missed in childhood or receiving routine recommended vaccine boosters. In 2015, 14.1 million cases of vaccine-preventable diseases were attributed to unvaccinated adults. To protect against infectious diseases, it's a good idea for adults to make sure that their vaccines are up to date and that they have received all recommended vaccine boosters.

Vaccine-preventable adult diseases include the following:

- Chicken pox (varicella)
- Diphtheria
- Flu (influenza)
- Hepatitis A
- Hepatitis B

- Human papillomavirus (HPV)
- Measles
- Meningococcal disease
- Mumps
- Pneumococcal disease
- Rubella
- Shingles (zoster)
- Tetanus
- Whooping cough (pertussis)

Question: What are antibiotics, and how do they work?

Answer: An antibiotic is any substance that inhibits the growth and replication of a bacterium or kills it outright. A type of antimicrobial, an antibiotic is designed to target bacterial infections in or on the body. Although scientists did not discover that infections were caused by bacteria until the late 1800s, different forms of antibiotics have been used to treat infections for thousands of years.

Early civilizations used compounds found in nature, such as certain plants and molds, to treat infections. Today, most antibiotics are produced in laboratories, although scientists still use natural compounds as a basis for their research.

Ukrainian-born Jewish American Nobel Prize-winning microbiologist, biochemist, and inventor Selman Waksman (1888–1973) is credited with coining the term *antibiotics* in 1942 to describe antibacterials that were derived from other living organisms.

Antibiotics target bacteria by either preventing the bacteria from reproducing or by killing the bacteria. Some antibiotics are developed to be highly specialized against certain types of bacteria. Others are broad-spectrum antibiotics, intended to work against a wide range of bacteria.

Question: Are antibiotics an effective treatment for infectious diseases?

Answer: Antibiotics work against bacteria and are an effective treatment for bacterial infections, but they cannot kill viruses and, therefore, cannot be used to treat viral infections—including colds and flu.

If a bacterium is the cause of an infectious disease, such as bacterial pneumonia, antibiotics will usually kill the bacteria and end the infection.

Question: What are antiviral drugs, and how are they used to treat infectious diseases?

Answer: While antibiotics can work only against bacteria, infectious diseases caused by viruses can be treated with antiviral medications, which fight the infection by either limiting the virus's ability to reproduce or by strengthening the body's immune response to the invading infection.

Antiviral drugs come in a variety of forms, including pills, liquid, inhaled powder, and intravenous solution. There are antiviral drugs to treat a number of viruses that cause infectious diseases, including hepatitis B, HIV/AIDS, and influenza.

Question: What does an allergy to eggs have to do with whether you can receive certain vaccines?

Answer: There are currently four vaccines that are cultured either in eggs or in chick embryos, which means the final vaccine product contains a small amount of egg protein. Therefore, people who are allergic to eggs could experience an allergic reaction to certain vaccines.

These are the four vaccines that contain egg protein:

- Influenza
- Measles, mumps, rubella (MMR)
- Rabies
- Yellow fever

Only two of these vaccines, influenza and MMR, are recommended to be administered to all children younger than two, a time when egg allergies are most common. But even among these four vaccines, the amount of egg protein varies, making some of them safer than others.

For instance, the MMR vaccine, which is typically given twice in childhood, is cultured in chicken embryos and contains only trace amounts of egg protein. Researchers have not found that children experience an allergic reaction to the vaccine, so it is considered safe even for people who have severe egg allergies.

Almost all of the influenza vaccines on the market are cultured in chicken eggs. Although the CDC recommends that everyone age six months and older receive an annual flu shot, they recommend that children with egg allergies be closely monitored by a physician for allergic reactions following the vaccine. At this time, two flu vaccines do not use chicken eggs in manufacturing.

Rabies is a zoonotic disease that, although rare, can lead to death if left untreated. A variety of rabies vaccines on the market can be administered after exposure to the rabies virus. Like the MMR vaccine, most of the vaccines for rabies are cultured in chicken embryos, but unlike the MMR vaccine, they are not considered safe for people who have severe allergies to egg protein. One vaccine, however, is not cultured in egg embryos, making it safe for people who are allergic to egg protein.

Yellow fever is a mosquito-borne illness common in parts of South America and Africa. This illness has a high mortality rate, so travelers to parts of the world where yellow fever is prevalent are advised to receive the yellow fever vaccine prior to the trip. But because the yellow fever vaccine is cultured in eggs, a doctor may recommend that a person with a history of severe egg-allergic reactions be referred to an allergist for consideration of allergy desensitization. If allergy desensitization is not possible, it may be possible to request a medical waiver for entry into a country requiring the vaccine. A person with a mild egg allergy may be able to receive the vaccine or have the vaccine allergy tested before it is administered.

Question: Which infectious diseases were much more common before vaccines were developed for them?

Answer: Because they have greatly benefited from childhood vaccinations, people born in the preceding few decades may be unaware of just how many diseases were once a serious public health concern.

The development of these vaccines—many of which protect against common childhood diseases—has greatly reduced or eliminated the number of cases of fourteen diseases in the United States:

- Chicken pox
- Diphtheria
- Hepatitis A
- Hepatitis B
- Hib (Haemophilus influenzae type b)
- Influenza
- Measles
- Mumps
- Pneumococcal disease
- Polio
- Rotavirus
- Rubella
- Tetanus
- Whooping cough (pertussis)

Question: **Does every infectious disease have a vaccine?**

Answer: Vaccines are one of humankind's greatest inventions. They have transformed the way people live and have also extended our life expectancy. In England during the seventeenth century, one third of all children died before the age of fifteen, often due to infectious diseases. Today that number is less than 1 percent—due in large part to the contributions of vaccine science.

So the good news is that many of the deadliest infectious diseases in the world have a vaccine. Unfortunately, not only do some diseases lack an effective vaccine, the vaccines we do have offer varying degrees of protection against disease. Ebola, for instance, now has a vaccine that is almost 100 percent effective in its protection, while the annual seasonal influenza vaccine ranges in effectiveness from year to year.

Many of the diseases that do not yet have a vaccine are considered neglected tropical diseases (NTDs) and are most prevalent in poor populations of economically underdeveloped countries.

Here are a few of the most serious infectious diseases that don't yet have a vaccine:

- Chagas disease (American trypanosomiasis)
- Chikungunya
- Cytomegalovirus
- Dengue
- HIV/AIDS
- Hookworm infection
- Leishmaniasis
- Malaria
- Respiratory syncytial virus
- Schistosomiasis (bilharziasis)

Question: **Why are some vaccines more effective than others? And what are booster shots?**

Answer: Vaccines work to provide immunity against disease, and overall the effectiveness of most vaccines is great. But not every vaccine provides 100 percent immunity. For instance, the inactivated polio vaccine provides 99 percent immunity against the disease after three doses.

Although some vaccines, such as the Ebola virus vaccine, provide lifelong immunity with a single dose, other vaccines require one or more booster shots to provide a continuously high level of immunity. Some booster shots are given infrequently, such as the tetanus booster, which is recommended every ten years. Other vaccines require more frequent booster shots, such as the annual flu vaccine.

Scientists don't completely understand why immunity varies with different vaccines. Because vaccines are designed to generate an immune response, the level of immunity achieved can vary, depending on how a person's immune system responds to the vaccine. Another variable is that not every person develops immunity to a given vaccine. In fact, the recommended childhood vaccines provide immunity in only 85 to 95 percent of the children who receive them. This is another example of the importance of herd immunity.

Research suggests that consistent immunity against a disease may be related to a combination of factors, including the speed of the disease's progression throughout the body and the immune system's ability to quickly recognize the pathogen. In a slow-moving infection, the immune system has more time to recognize and respond to the infection, and booster vaccines are generally not required to maintain immunity.

The ability of the immune system to respond to detected pathogens is called immunological memory. In a rapidly progressing disease, the body's immune system may not be able to respond fast enough to stave off infection. A booster shot can help ramp up the body's immunological memory so that the immune system can respond quickly to a pathogen.

Question: **Where did whooping cough get its name?**

Answer: Pertussis is more commonly referred to as *whooping cough.* It is a highly contagious respiratory disease caused by bacterial infection of the respiratory tract. The bacterium that causes whooping cough is *Bordatella pertussis.*

Pertussis causes uncontrollable, painful coughing, which makes it difficult for the person to breathe. The disease takes its name from the deep, gasping breaths that cause a "whoop" sound when a person (usually a child) has a violent bout of coughing.

Not everyone who has pertussis makes the distinct whooping sound associated with the disease, and the presence (or lack) of a "whoop" cough cannot be used to make a diagnosis.

Anyone can get whooping cough, and the best way to prevent this illness is to be vaccinated against it. For maximum protection from whooping cough, the CDC's immunization schedule for infants and young children recommends five shots of the DTaP vaccine, starting at two months of age. Babies younger than one year old are at the highest risk of becoming seriously ill if they get whooping cough because they haven't yet been fully vaccinated. For this reason, it's recommended that pregnant women be vaccinated against whooping cough in their third trimester and that other adults in close contact with a young infant be up to date on their own whooping cough vaccine.

Question: How do you know when you have an infectious disease? Do all infectious diseases have similar symptoms?

Answer: Because different infectious diseases are caused by different agents, including bacteria, viruses, fungi, and parasites, their characteristics can vary dramatically from one infectious disease to the next. That said, several symptoms are common to many infectious diseases. These include the following:

- Cough
- Diarrhea
- Fatigue
- Fever
- Muscle aches

Diagnosis of an infectious disease requires a medical exam and laboratory tests. A person who experiences any of the following should seek medical attention:

- Trouble breathing
- Coughing for more than a week
- Severe headache accompanied by fever
- Unexplained rash or swelling
- Sudden vision problems
- Animal bite (including from a domestic animal)

CHAPTER 2

OUTBREAKS, EPIDEMICS, AND PANDEMICS

How Diseases Affect Large Populations

Question: What does "level of disease" mean?

Answer: In the study of epidemiology, the level of disease reflects the amount of a particular infectious disease in a community. The level of disease can and does change, based on a number of factors. The following list describes various levels of disease as defined by the CDC:

Endemic: a disease that has a constant presence or prevalence in a particular geographic area.

Sporadic: a disease that occurs infrequently and irregularly.

Hyperendemic: a disease that has a persistent and high level of occurrence in a geographic area.

Epidemic: the situation when the level of disease in a population rises, unexpectedly and often rapidly, above the usual anticipated level.

Outbreak: an epidemic, usually in a limited geographic area.

Cluster: an aggregation of infectious disease cases grouped in place and time that are believed to be greater than the number of cases expected—even though the expected number of cases may be unknown.

Pandemic: an epidemic that has spread across several countries or continents, affecting a large number of people.

Question: What's the difference between an epidemic and a pandemic?

Answer: An epidemic occurs when there is a sudden and unexpected increase in the number of cases of an infectious disease within a specific population or geographic region. If the United States, or even a particular geographic region within the country, experienced a sudden uptick in the number of flu cases during a flu season, the flu would be labeled an epidemic.

The term *pandemic* describes the spread of an infectious disease across many countries and populations. There aren't any specific guidelines for how many countries must be affected or how many people must contract the disease in order for it to be labeled a pandemic. Instead, the spread of a disease is labeled a pandemic if there is an expectation that everyone could be exposed.

The easiest way to remember the difference between an epidemic and a pandemic is to remember that the P in *pandemic* stands for *passport*. A pandemic is an epidemic that can travel anywhere, and the assumption is that everyone can be exposed.

Question: **How is a cluster different from an outbreak?**

Answer: Like an infectious disease epidemic, an outbreak is the rise in the number of cases of an infectious disease in excess of what is normally anticipated for that particular disease. The terms *outbreak* and *epidemic* are often used interchangeably to mean the same thing, but an outbreak is the sudden increase in the number of cases of an infectious disease in a localized geographic area, such as a town, or in a closed institution, such as a school or prison.

The CDC defines an outbreak as three or more cases of an infectious disease, but the actual number can vary depending on the disease. In fact, an outbreak can be declared with just a single case of a rare infectious disease, such as foodborne botulism, or a disease caused by a bioterrorism agent, such as anthrax, which may have serious public health implications.

A cluster is the number of cases of an infectious disease grouped in place and time, regardless of whether the number of cases is greater than expected for that area. It is important for researchers to determine whether a cluster of cases is an outbreak caused by a common infectious disease or the cases are somehow unrelated.

Question: **What causes an epidemic?**

Answer: In order for an infectious disease to reach epidemic level, an infectious agent, or pathogen, must be present, in addition to an adequate number of susceptible hosts so that the agent can be passed from a source to the susceptible hosts.

An infectious disease epidemic may result from several factors, including these:

- A recent increase in the amount or virulence of the infectious agent
- The introduction of an emerging infectious agent into a setting where it has not previously existed
- A mode of transmission that allows for more susceptible hosts to be exposed to the infectious agent
- A change in the ecology of the host population

- A genetic change in the infectious agent
- An increase in host exposure to the infectious agent or the introduction of the infectious agent through new portals of entry

Question: What is a zoonotic disease?

Answer: A zoonotic disease, or zoonosis, is a disease that typically exists in animals or insects and can be transmitted to humans. Like any other infectious disease, a zoonotic disease can be caused by bacteria, fungi, parasites, or viruses. A zoonotic disease, such as malaria or Lyme disease, can be spread by insects, such as mosquitoes (in the case of malaria) or ticks (in the case of Lyme disease).

The terms *zoonotic* and *zoonosis* do not refer to zoos or zoo animals specifically. Places where people come into contact with animals—such as fairs, petting zoos, or live animal exhibits—can be a source of zoonotic disease.

Zoonotic diseases are among the most common types of infectious disease. There are several ways zoonotic diseases can spread, including the following:

- Breathing in contaminated respiratory droplets
- Eating contaminated food, such as meat or produce
- Coming into close contact with an infected animal or something the animal has touched
- Receiving bites from insects, such as mosquitoes, fleas, or ticks

Perhaps the best-known example of a zoonotic disease is rabies. This viral illness is transmitted through the saliva of an infected animal. Rabies transmission can occur from animal to animal or from animal to human through an animal bite or through the animal's saliva coming into contact with an open wound or the mucous membranes of another animal or a human.

Examples of zoonotic diseases include the following:

- Animal flu
- Anthrax
- Bird flu
- Bovine tuberculosis
- Brucellosis
- Campylobacter infection
- Cat scratch fever
- Cryptosporidiosis
- Cysticercosis
- Dengue fever
- Ebola
- Encephalitis from ticks
- Enzootic abortion
- Erysipeloid
- Fish tank granuloma
- Giardiasis
- Glanders
- Hemorrhagic colitis
- Hepatitis E
- Hydatid disease
- Leptospirosis
- Listeria infection
- Louping ill virus
- Lyme disease
- Lymphocytic choriomeningitis
- Malaria
- Orf infection
- Parrot fever
- Pasteurellosis
- Plague
- Q fever
- Rabies
- Rat-bite fever
- Ringworm

- Rocky Mountain spotted fever
- *Salmonella* and *E. coli* infections
- Streptococcal sepsis
- Swine flu
- Toxocariasis
- Toxoplasmosis
- Trichinellosis
- Tularemia
- West Nile virus
- Zoonotic diphtheria

Question: **How is global warming affecting the spread of infectious diseases?**

Answer: Scientists are concerned that global warming may do more than cause extreme weather changes in the coming years—it could also cause the significant spread of old and new infectious diseases in places that were previously considered safe.

As average temperatures increase in temperate climates, the risk of infectious diseases spreading also increases because insects find new habitats farther north. Diseases, such as mosquito-borne Zika virus and tick-borne Lyme disease, could spread to new areas due to more hospitable environmental factors provided by longer, warmer summers. Other global warming issues, such as flooding and drought, can contribute to the spread of disease, as mosquitoes breed in collected rainwater and cholera bacteria spread in contaminated water.

Similarly, the melting of the Arctic's permafrost could allow the release of ancient pathogens that have been frozen in the ice for centuries. We are already seeing the potential disease risks associated with melting permafrost (See "What is a zombie pathogen?" on page 46.)

(See "What is a zombie pathogen?" on page 46.)

Question: What is a zombie pathogen?

Answer: Although it sounds like something out of a horror movie, zombie pathogens are becoming increasingly real concerns for researchers studying the thawing of the Arctic's permafrost. These ancient pathogens include bacteria and viruses that have been preserved in the frozen ground or frozen animal carcasses that could potentially come back to life as the permafrost thaws due to global warming.

Although the chance of infectious diseases becoming reanimated like a fictional zombie is believed to be small, the 2016 anthrax outbreak in Siberia demonstrates that it isn't entirely impossible. This outbreak killed more than two thousand reindeer, caused dozens of people to be hospitalized, and resulted in the death of a twelve-year-old boy. The outbreak occurred following an unseasonably warm summer that thawed the soil where a seventy-five-year-old reindeer carcass had been buried.

In a similar incident in 2017, teacher Zac Peterson was assisting archaeologists in the excavation of an eight-hundred-year-old log cabin above the Arctic Circle on the northern coast of Alaska. Toward the end of the excavation, Peterson developed a skin infection that was diagnosed as seal finger—a bacterial infection so named because it is contracted by hunters who have handled the body parts of infected seals. The only seals Peterson had come in contact with on his trip were those found in the excavated log cabin—and they had been frozen in perma-frost for decades.

Question: Are infectious diseases the top cause of death in the world?

Answer: According to the most recent World Health Organization statistics from 2016, infectious diseases hold three of the top ten causes of death globally. These diseases are as follows:

- Lower respiratory infections (3 million deaths)
- Diarrheal diseases (1.4 million deaths)
- Tuberculosis (1.3 million deaths)

Lower respiratory infections rank fourth in leading causes of global deaths, behind heart disease, stroke, and chronic obstructive pulmonary disease (COPD).

Among low-income countries, five infectious diseases—lower respiratory infections, diarrheal diseases, HIV/AIDS, malaria, and tuberculosis—are among the top ten causes of death, with lower respiratory infections and diarrheal diseases in the top two spots. In contrast, only lower respiratory infections rank in the top ten causes of death in high-income countries.

Question: What is public health surveillance, and why do we track the number of deaths caused by infectious diseases?

Answer: Public health surveillance is the systematic collection, analysis, and interpretation of health data. Collecting the data allows epidemiologists to calculate the incidence (number of new cases reported throughout a specified time period), prevalence (number of cases at one specific time), hospitalizations, and deaths attributed to an infectious disease. This information allows public health officials to formulate, implement, and evaluate public health plans.

Tracking how and where people die provides important data for assessing how well a country's health system is working. These data allow public health authorities to focus their efforts where they are most needed.

Question: **What have been the deadliest pandemics in human history?**

Answer: Humanity has lived with infectious diseases since the dawn of time. And, as science advances, we continue to learn about the diseases that our ancestors lived with—and died from.

The true impact of any infectious disease cannot be measured by the number of people who succumb to the disease. Likewise, the number of deaths that occur during an epidemic or pandemic cannot tell us the long-lasting and far-reaching effects of those catastrophic events. But these are the pandemics whose death tolls mark them as some of the most significant events in human history:

ANTONINE PLAGUE (165–180 CE)
Death toll: 5 million

Cause: Unknown

PLAGUE OF JUSTINIAN (541–49 CE)

Death toll: 25–100 million

Cause: Bubonic plague

BLACK DEATH (1346–53)

Death toll: 75–200 million

Cause: Bubonic plague

THIRD CHOLERA PANDEMIC (1852–60)

Death toll: 1 million

Cause: Cholera

FLU PANDEMIC (1889–90)

(referred to as the Asiatic flu or the Russian flu)

Death toll: 1 million

Cause: Influenza

1918 FLU PANDEMIC (1918–20)

Death toll: 20–50 million

Cause: Influenza

ASIAN FLU (1956–58)

Death toll: 2 million

Cause: Influenza

FLU PANDEMIC (1968)

(referred to as the Hong Kong flu)

Death toll: 1 million

Cause: Influenza

HIV/AIDS PANDEMIC (AT ITS PEAK, 2005–2012)

Death toll: 36 million

Cause: HIV/AIDS

Question: Could a pandemic on the scale of the Black Death ever happen again?

Answer: The short answer is no, we won't see another Black Death in human history. Medical and scientific advances, as well as modern sanitation practices, stronger immunity, and better nutrition make it very unlikely that the world could experience a naturally occurring plague outbreak on the scale of the Black Death pandemic of the fourteenth century.

Of course, the key phrase is "naturally occurring." Weaponizing plague, particularly the pneumonic form of plague, could be an effective method of biological warfare, although it still seems doubtful that it could rival the deadliest pandemic in recorded history.

Question: What are the phases of a pandemic?

Answer: Both the World Health Organization (WHO) and the Centers for Disease Control and Prevention (CDC) have guidelines that advise officials on how to proceed during an influenza pandemic. These guidelines are also being used for the COVID-19 pandemic.

The WHO's pandemic alert system identifies six phases of an influenza pandemic. This phased system was developed in 1999 and revised in 2005 and 2009, offering global guidelines to assist countries in preparing for and responding to a pandemic.

The six phases of the WHO's pandemic alert system:

- **Phase 1:** There have been no reported cases of infection in humans as a result of an influenza virus circulating in animals.

- **Phase 2:** An animal virus circulating in animals (wild or domestic) has been reported to be the cause of infection in humans. The virus is considered a potential pandemic threat.

- **Phase 3:** Sporadic or small clusters of disease have been reported, but any human-to-human transmission has not been sufficient to cause a community-level outbreak.

- **Phase 4:** Community-level outbreaks have been reported as a result of human-to-human transmission.

- **Phase 5:** The same virus has caused sustained community-level outbreaks in two or more countries located in one WHO region.

- **Phase 6:** As well as reaching the Phase 5 criteria, the same virus has also caused sustained community-level outbreaks in at least one other country in a different WHO region.

In addition to the six phases, the WHO has designated two periods that follow a pandemic:

- **Postpeak period:** In most countries with adequate health surveillance measures, pandemic levels of influenza have dropped below peak levels.

- **Postpandemic period:** In most countries with adequate health surveillance measures, levels of influenza activity have dropped to the level of seasonal influenza.

The WHO's guidelines include action plans that coincide with each of the pandemic phases. The main actions for each pandemic phase include the following:

- Planning and coordination
- Situation monitoring and assessment
- Communications
- Reducing the spread of disease
- Continuity of health care provision

The CDC has a complementary influenza pandemic guideline used by the United States called the Pandemic Intervals Framework (PIF). The PIF describes the progression of an influenza pandemic through six intervals that align with the WHO's pandemic phases:

1. Investigation of novel influenza virus infections in humans

2. Recognition that the infections could spread farther and faster

3. Initiation of a pandemic wave

4. Acceleration of a pandemic wave

5. Deceleration of a pandemic wave

6. Preparation for future pandemic waves

Each of the CDC's pandemic intervals in this framework offers recommendations regarding risk assessment, decision making, and action items for the United States.

Question: How do experts determine when a pandemic is over? What is the difference between a medical end and a social end to a pandemic?

Answer: Although infectious disease pandemics are often compared to wars in terms of the mortality rate, unlike a war, a pandemic does not have a hard and fast end point. Because the disease that is causing a pandemic may be new to the population it is affecting, or is caused by an entirely new (novel) virus (such as COVID-19), there is no single pandemic model that works when it comes to declaring an end to a pandemic.

Historically, there have been two types of pandemic endings: the medical ending and the social ending. The medical end of a pandemic is declared when herd immunity is achieved, either through vaccination or by a large enough percentage of the population—at least 70 percent—having been compromised by the disease.

Before a pandemic can end, the rates of disease activity and mortality must fall below the baseline for the disease— and remain there for a period. There is no set amount of time for how long this dormancy period must last before the pandemic is declared over because every disease is different and a number of variables must be considered. Outbreaks and additional disease waves can occur, and certain regional areas can become hot spots for new incidences of disease, especially in the absence of a vaccine or without proper surveillance.

The social end of a pandemic occurs when the population's fear of the disease subsides. This generally doesn't occur until after the medical end of the pandemic, when the risk of disease has been reduced due to vaccination or herd immunity. But a social end to a pandemic can occur before the medical end if a population becomes tired of living in crisis mode and instead learns to live with the disease and its potential consequences. This social end may result in a sense of normalcy among members of the population, but it does not signal a medical end—which means disease numbers can continue to spike and the disease can continue to linger in the population.

Question: What are biological weapons, and how are they used?

Answer: Biological weapons are also called bioweapons or biological warfare agents. They are intentionally produced and released microorganisms, such as bacteria, fungi, viruses, or other toxins, in order to cause disease and death in humans, animals, or plants. The use of biological agents as a weapon is bioterrorism.

Biological weapons belong to the class of weapons known as weapons of mass destruction, which also includes chemical, nuclear, and radiological weapons. The use of biological agents could cause public health issues by spreading quickly and being difficult to contain, or could even lead to an infectious disease epidemic.

A number of agents and diseases can be used as biological weapons or in bioterrorism events, and the CDC categorizes them based on their level of priority.

CATEGORY A

High-priority agents include microorganisms that pose a risk to national security. These agents can be easily spread among a population or transmitted from person to person. They also could result in high mortality rates and could cause public panic or have a major impact on public health. Special actions by government and public health officials are needed to prepare for these agents. High-priority agents and diseases include these:

- Anthrax
- Plague
- Botulism
- Smallpox

- Tularemia
- Viral hemorrhagic fevers, including Ebola, Marburg, Lassa, and Machupo

CATEGORY B

The second-highest priority agents are those that are moderately easy to circulate among a population and could result in moderate levels of sickness, with low mortality rates. These agents require specific enhanced disease surveillance to assure preparedness. Second-highest priority agents include the following:

- Brucellosis
- Epsilon toxin of *Clostridium perfringens*
- Food safety threats, such as *Salmonella*, *E. coli*, or *Shigella*
- Glanders
- Melioidosis
- Psittacosis

- Q fever
- Ricin toxin
- *Staphylococcal enterotoxin* B
- Typhus fever
- Viral encephalitis
- Water safety threats

CATEGORY C

The third-highest priority agents are emerging pathogens that could be engineered in the future. Their potential as biological weapons is due to their availability, ease of production and dissemination, and potential for causing a major health impact, with high illness and death rates. These third-highest priority agents include emerging infectious diseases such as these:

- Hantavirus
- Nipah virus

Question: Have biological weapons ever been used?

Answer: Biological warfare may seem like something out of a political thriller or a summer blockbuster film, but biological weapons have a long and deadly history that predates the development of germ theory by a few thousand years. Human and animal bodies—infected with a variety of infectious diseases, from plague to rabies—have been used against enemies.

Here are a few examples of the diabolical ways infectious diseases have been weaponized throughout history:

- **1155**: On a campaign of conquest in Italy, Holy Roman Emperor Frederick Barbarossa used human corpses to poison the well water.

- **1346**: During the Siege of Caffa, Mongol combatants hurled the bodies of plague victims over the walls of this Crimean city.

- **1495**: The Spanish mixed the blood of leprosy patients with wine and then sold it to the French.

- **1650**: Polish general Casimir Siemienowicz had clay or glass balls filled with the saliva of rabid dogs and catapulted at enemies.

- **1763**: The British distributed blankets from smallpox patients to Native Americans.

- **1797**: Napoleon exacerbated the spread of malaria by flooding the plains around Mantua, Italy.

- **1863**: Confederates sold the clothing of yellow fever and smallpox patients to Union troops.

Louis Pasteur's and Robert Koch's work in the discipline of microbiology set the stage for the potential abuse of manufactured biological agents.

Two international treaties were drafted in the twentieth century with the goal of preventing bioterrorism: the Geneva Protocol of 1925 and the Biological Weapons Convention of 1972. Unfortunately, these good faith declarations offered no means of controlling the research, production, or use of such biological weapons.

The twentieth and early twenty-first centuries have seen a variety of incidents involving the weaponization of biological agents. Today, the World Health Organization works with governments concerned about bioterrorism to prepare for the possibility of such an event.

Question: What is the Biological Weapons Convention?

Answer: The Biological Weapons Convention (BWC) is an international treaty that makes biological arms illegal. It was discussed and negotiated in the United Nations' disarmament forum beginning in 1969, it opened for signing on April 10, 1972, and it entered into force on March 26, 1975.

The BWC bans the development, stockpiling, acquisition, retention, or production of biological agents or toxins of the types and in the quantities that cannot be justified for pro-phylactic, protective, or peaceful purposes. Also banned in the BWC are the equipment, weapons, and vehicles designed for use during armed conflict with such agents or toxins. Assisting with or transferring such agents, toxins, equipment, weapons, or vehicles are also prohibited, and the BWC requires the destruction, or diversion to peaceful purposes, of these items.

The BWC does not ban the use of biological or toxin weapons, but reaffirms the 1925 Geneva Protocol, which prohibits such use. There is also no ban on biodefense programs.

As of August 2019, 183 states-parties have ratified or acceded to the BWC.

Question: **What was the earliest use of biological warfare?**

Answer: Historical documents suggest that biological weapons may have been used with intention more than 3,300 years ago.

The texts, dating to the fourteenth century BCE in the Middle East, suggest that the Hittites, a people of Bronze Age Anatolia whose empire stretched from modern-day Turkey to northern Syria, weaponized rams infected with tularemia, a bacterial infection. It is believed that the animals were driven into enemy lands with the intention of causing the spread of disease.

Although there isn't enough evidence to establish the success of this method, a "Hittite plague" is documented in the ancient texts. Tularemia seems to have worked against the Hittites as well. They stole infected animals during attacks on their enemies and later became sick themselves.

Tularemia still exists in the modern era and is still considered a potential bioterror threat. Also known as rabbit fever, tularemia is a zoonotic disease that can be passed to humans from animals such as rabbits or sheep. The method of transmission is most often through insects such as ticks. Antibiotics can prevent tularemia from becoming fatal. Untreated cases have a mortality rate of around 15 percent.

Question: **Which country was the first to use biological and chemical weapons of mass destruction in the modern era?**

Answer: During World War I, Germany was the first country to use both biological and chemical weapons of mass destruction.

Engaging in small-scale covert operations, the German army had minimal success with infecting animals and animal feed with two biological agents, anthrax and glanders. During the war, there were reports that the Germans intended to ship infected animals and animal feed to the United States and other countries.

Germany was also accused of attempting to spread cholera in Italy and plague in St. Petersburg, Russia. Despite the evidence that pointed to Germany having an active biological warfare program during the war, German officials denied the allegations.

The Geneva Protocol of 1925 was created in response to the use of poisonous gas by both sides in the conflict. Commercial chemicals such as chlorine, phosgene, and mustard gas were used as weapons, causing around 100,000 deaths as a result.

Although biological weapons had been only minimally effective during the war, the title of the treaty was the "Protocol for the Prohibition of the Use in War of Asphyxiating, Poisonous or Other Gases and of Bacteriological Methods of Warfare." At the time, viruses were not yet being differentiated from bacteria, which is why they were not specifically addressed.

Initially signed by 108 nations, the Geneva Protocol made no provisions for verifying the compliance of the countries that signed the agreement, making it unenforceable. Despite the United States being an initial supporter of the Geneva Protocol, the US military and American Chemical Society were not in favor of it and lobbied against it. As a result, the US Senate did not ratify the Geneva Protocol until 1975.

Question: Who was Shirō Ishii, and what was his role in the development of biological weapons?

Answer: Shirō Ishii (1892–1959) was a Japanese micro-biologist and medical officer. He was also one of the most notorious war criminals in modern history.

The United States wasn't the only world power that did not sign the Geneva Protocol of 1925—Japan also declined to sign the agreement. In fact, it was the Geneva Protocol that caused Shirō Ishii to turn his focus to the use of biological weapons in warfare. He was in favor of Japan creating a bacteriological weapons program, urging that biological weapons would not have been banned by the protocol if they weren't highly effective.

Although the United States and Great Britain tested biological weapons on animals during World War II, human tests were unethical and therefore prohibited. Ishii had no such limitations placed on his testing and, over a span of several years, used human test subjects, with horrific results.

In 1932, the Japanese government put Ishii in charge of a testing and production facility in Manchuria, a province in China that the Japanese had previously invaded. Guided by a single-minded focus to defeat Japan's enemies at any cost, Ishii set about creating a massive secret facility that became known as Unit 731. Completed in 1940, Unit 731 had more than three thousand people on staff—all dedicated to Ishii's singular cause.

Over the next five years, Ishii and his team used Chinese prisoners as test subjects to measure the effects on humans of breathing, consuming, and receiving injections of a variety of virulent disease agents. Many of Unit 731's records were destroyed following its dissolution at the end of the war in 1945, but enough documentation remains to suggest that Ishii's work was responsible for the deaths of thousands of Chinese, as well as contributing to hundreds of deaths of Russian and Allied prisoners of war.

Among the deadly pathogens that Ishii unleashed on prisoners at Unit 731 were anthrax, botulism, gas gangrene, plague, and smallpox. He also gave the Japanese army biological pathogens for battlefield use, including cholera, dysentery bacteria, plague, and typhoid, making it possible for them to drop contaminated grain from airplanes, contaminate water supplies, and release disease-carrying fleas on their enemies.

During the US occupation of Japan at the end of World War II, the Japanese transferred Shirō Ishii to the United States at the order of US occupation forces. During interrogation, Ishii agreed to give the United States information about his biological weapons program in exchange for immunity for his substantial war crimes. Interested in learning the details of Ishii's work with biological weapons for their own biological warfare program, the US military sought and obtained approval from the US government for Ishii's immunity, as well as the immunity of Unit 731.

Although what information Ishii provided proved to be of little value to the United States, Ishii's immunity was nonetheless secured, and his work developing and testing biological weapons was not brought up in the course of the Japanese war crimes trials. Despite being responsible for an untold number of deaths through the use of disease pathogens, Ishii died a free man in Japan in 1959.

Question: Why do samples of smallpox still exist—and will they ever be destroyed?

Answer: Smallpox is an ancient disease caused by the variola virus. This highly contagious disease existed for at least three thousand years and was once a global scourge. It killed more people than all other contagious diseases combined. In the twentieth century alone, smallpox killed an estimated 300 million people.

Smallpox was eradicated in 1980 through a worldwide immunization program, one of modern medicine's greatest success stories. In the last years of the disease, all cases of smallpox were carefully identified and patients' contacts were traced to ensure everyone had been vaccinated. It was a long, complex process, but it worked. Today, there is no evidence of smallpox occurring naturally anywhere in the world. And yet there are still small quantities of smallpox in existence.

After smallpox was officially declared eradicated, most of the remaining stocks of variola virus were destroyed—but small amounts of the virus have been saved. These samples have been preserved for research and experimentation and are stored in liquid nitrogen vials in two research laboratories: the US Centers for Disease Control and Prevention in Atlanta, Georgia, and the State Research Centre of Virology and Biotechnology in the Siberian city of Novosibirsk, Russia. Their location is public knowledge, although the exact rooms and freezers in which they are stored are kept secret.

The World Health Organization (WHO) has decided the preserved stocks will be destroyed once improved vaccines and countermeasures have been developed to fight the disease in the event it reemerges through a lab accident or bioterrorism event. In 1999, the WHO Advisory Committee on Variola Virus Research was formed to oversee the research, and a yearly report is made to the WHO's decision-making body, the World Health Assembly.

So far, a decision on when to destroy the remaining smallpox stocks has been delayed, with scientists, scholars, and ethicists continuing to debate the need for their existence—and how close we are to reaching the goals that would allow us to destroy the samples.

CHAPTER 3

EARLY HISTORY OF INFECTIOUS DISEASES

Pestilence and Plague Doctors, Scourges and Sanatoriums—How Our Ancestors Lived with Disease

Question: Who was the first person to recognize that infectious diseases can be transmitted from person to person?

Answer: When plague swept through Athens, Greece, between 430 and 427 BCE, it laid the groundwork for further understanding of infectious diseases and how they are spread. The plague struck during the second year of the Peloponnesian War (431–404 BCE) and killed an estimated seventy-five thousand to one hundred thousand people. It is possible that Greek statesman, general, and orator Pericles may have helped facilitate the rapid spread of the disease throughout the population of Athens by calling for his people to withdraw behind the protective walls of the city as the war began to escalate.

In writing *History of the Peloponnesian War*, Athenian historian and general Thucydides included his detailed account of the Plague of Athens. His insights have given historians and researchers valuable information about the epidemiology of the plague that killed so many Athenians. Although there is no contemporary pathogen that manifests exactly as Thucydides describes in his notes, some contemporary researchers believe that Athens might have experienced an outbreak of smallpox.

Thucydides has been called the father of scientific history because he claimed to believe in applying rigid standards of impartiality and evidence-gathering and eschewed explanations of divine intervention. Demonstrating a keen understanding of cause and effect, he kept meticulous notes about how he believed the disease was being transmitted from person to person. Thucydides observed that many of the people who fell victim to illness lived in the most densely populated areas of Athens, and that doctors and healers who cared for the sick and dying were themselves likely to die from the plague. He also noted how the disease was passed between groups of Athenian soldiers as they went to and came from the front lines of battle, leading him to deduce that it was possible for the disease to be transmitted.

Thucydides's shrewd analyses of how the disease spread throughout the population of Athens is particularly noteworthy for his era. At the time, the medical theory was that infectious disease was spread by miasma, an airborne poison. Miasma was presumed to be caused by anything from the weather to rotting animal flesh to angry gods. Thucydides not only gave us the sole known first-person account of the Plague of Athens, but he also survived the disease himself.

Question: Who was Galen, and what is miasma theory?

Answer: *Miasma* is a term used to describe a poisonous vapor ("bad air" or "night air") that was once believed to cause illness and disease and was said to have a disgusting odor. The obsolete miasma theory of disease (also called miasmatic theory) dates as far back as ancient Greece in the fourth or fifth century BCE and was widely accepted in Europe and China. At the time, the Greek physician Hippocrates believed that disease was caused by an imbalance of the four humors (yellow bile, black bile, phlegm, and blood) and that "bad air" was the cause of pestilence.

Hippocrates's humoral theory was expanded upon by other physicians, most notably Galen of Pergamon (129–216 CE), a celebrated Greco-Roman physician, writer, and philosopher, who hypothesized that a person's susceptibility to a disease could be traced to an imbalance of the four humors.

Galen's influence on medicine continued beyond the Middle Ages, with "bad air" being used as an explanation for why some people contracted plague and others did not. Owing to the importance of both Hippocrates and Galen, the miasma theory of contagion continued to be the dominant theory of disease until the mid-nineteenth century. When the Industrial Revolution began and poor air quality became the norm in cities, miasma was believed to cause the spread of cholera, notably in London and Paris in the 1850s.

Question: **What does the Bible say about plague and pestilence?**

The word *pestilence* comes from *pestis*, the Latin word meaning "plague." The words *pestilence* and *plague* are often used interchangeably in literature to refer to a variety of catastrophic ailments and events.

The terms *pestilence* and *plague* are mentioned several times in the Old Testament, the New Testament, and the Apocrypha. The ten Plagues of Egypt described in the book of Exodus were said to be ten divine disasters inflicted on the lands and people of Egypt to compel the pharaoh to free the Israelites. These are the Plagues of Egypt:

1. Water turned to blood

2. Frogs

3. Lice

4. Wild beasts

5. Pestilence

6. Skin disease

7. Fiery hail

8. Locusts

9. Darkness

10. Killing of the firstborn son

Contemporary researchers hypothesize that several of the Plagues of Egypt could actually be related to infectious diseases. The water turning to blood referenced in the first plague might be a red algae bloom, which can contaminate a body of water and cause illness in people and animals who either drink the polluted water, eat the contaminated fish or shellfish, or even breathe the aerosols around the polluted water.

The lice of the third plague has been interpreted in some translations to be fleas. In either case, both body lice and fleas can transmit *Yersinia pestis*, the pathogen that causes bubonic plague. The wild beasts of the fourth plague are interpreted by some theological scholars to mean flies, whose bites could have led to the skin disease of the sixth plague.

The fifth plague, livestock pestilence, is a highly contagious disease that killed off the Egyptians' livestock. Based on the description of how the disease ravaged animal herds, researchers believe the disease could have been rinderpest. This disease is thought to have originated in Asia and traveled to Egypt five thousand years ago via prehistoric cattle-trading routes. Rinderpest can travel quickly through livestock and has a mortality rate of around 80 percent.

The skin disease of the sixth plague might have been boils caused by *Staphylococcus aureus*, a bacterium found on the skin. It could also have been smallpox, which causes raised blisters and is believed to have been in Egypt at least three thousand years ago.

The tenth and final Plague of Egypt is the death of first-born sons. Some theories suggest it could be related back to the first plague. A body of water contaminated by a red algae bloom could release mycotoxins, which are naturally occurring toxins produced by certain fungi. These mycotoxins could have contaminated the grain crops of the Egyptians, causing the death of older boys, who perhaps were given the job of picking the mature grain.

Although Exodus has the most comprehensive references to plague and pestilence, it is not the only biblical text to describe some of the infectious diseases that have affected the world for thousands of years.

Revelation 6 of the book of Revelation references the Four Horsemen of the Apocalypse, who represent four devastating events preceding the second coming of Jesus Christ. In the New Revised Standard Version (NRSV) translation of the Bible, the fourth horseman is Death:

I looked and there was a pale green horse! Its rider's name was Death, and Hades followed with him; they were given authority over a fourth of the earth, to kill with sword, famine, and pestilence, and by the wild animals of the earth.

In modern use, *pestilence* has come to refer to any epidemic disease that is highly contagious and devastating, such as bubonic plague, which is transmitted by fleas from infected rodents, most often rats.

Question: **Who were plague doctors—and why did they wear a costume?**

Answer: Plague doctors were physicians hired by towns to treat people who had contracted bubonic plague. During plague epidemics, these doctors would treat everyone who was suspected to be infected with plague—both the wealthy and the poor could expect a visit from the plague doctor. These doctors were tasked with a variety of duties, from prescribing treatments and antidotes, to witnessing the signing of wills, to performing autopsies on patients who had succumbed to their illness.

The dark and ominous head-to-toe outfit worn by plague doctors is credited to Charles de Lorme (1584–1678), a physician who cared for many of Europe's royal families during the seventeenth century. In 1619, de Lorme modeled his protective plague costume on a soldier's suit of armor, in the belief that the outfit would protect the doctor from miasma, the "bad air" that was believed to cause disease. His plague costume consisted of a long leather or waxed-canvas coat over the top of a tucked-in shirt, breeches connected to boots, gloves, and a hat. The grim ensemble also included a wooden cane, with which a doctor could examine patients without touching them—or use it to push the plague-infected away.

The creepily comical plague mask is a distinctive relic from the era. At the time, it was believed that heavily scented flowers, perfumes, and incense could cleanse the air and protect the wearer from contracting the plague. De Lorme surmised that filling the long, beak-like plague mask with a similar concoction could offer protection by suffusing the air adequately before it reached the doctor's nose and lungs. Of course, bubonic plague wasn't actually spread by breathing in bad air. So it's possible that the full-coverage plague doctor costume did help to protect doctors, not from bad air, but from the true cause of plague—the bite of fleas from infected rats.

Question: **When was quarantining sick people first recognized as a way to halt the spread of disease?**

Answer: Quarantining people as a method of limiting the spread of disease dates back to the fourteenth century, when the Black Death was ravaging Europe. Quarantine started as a way of preventing plague epidemics in coastal cities.

The word *quarantine* comes from the Italian *quaranta giorni*, or "forty days." During the time of the Black Death, Venice was the first city to close its ports to incoming ships, requiring ships from infected ports to sit at anchor for forty days before landing.

Venice established island quarantines, known as *lazza-rettos*, to limit the spread of the plague and protect the city. The first quarantine island, Lazzaretto Vecchio, was founded in 1423, housing a hospital for the treatment of plague patients. In 1468, a second island, Lazaretto Nuovo, was established for inbound ships, allowing crews and cargo to be isolated and inspected before proceeding to the port city.

Question: **Was "Typhoid Mary" a real person?**

Answer: Mary Mallon (1869–1938) was an Irish-born cook and the first person in the United States to be iden-tified as a chronic, asymptomatic carrier of *Salmonella enterica serovar typhi*, the agent that causes typhoid fever. Although she appeared healthy, Mallon was still able to infect people through her job as a domestic cook in New York City in the late 1800s. In due course, the Health Department of New York City was able to identify Mallon as a carrier and eventually traced fifty-three cases of typhoid back to her and her job preparing and handling food.

Once public health officials in New York made the con-nection between Mallon and the transmission of typhoid, they attempted to restrict her employment to stop the spread of the disease. But Mallon refused to comply with their demands and continued to work in food service—all the while continuing to spread typhoid. Mallon was forcibly quarantined twice and spent more than three decades of her life in isolation. Eventually, she was ordered quaran-tined on one of the islands outside Manhattan, where she remained until her death.

During her lifetime, Mary Mallon became known as "Typhoid Mary," a name still used to refer to asymptomatic disease carriers. It is believed that Mallon's mother was infected with typhoid during pregnancy and that Mallon was born with typhoid. Researchers estimate that as many as 6 percent of people infected with *Salmonella typhi* become chronic, asymptomatic carriers like Mallon.

Question: **What were the three great plague pandemics?**

Answer: History has recorded three great plague pandemics, which occurred in the sixth century, the fourteenth century, and the late-nineteenth to the mid-twentieth centuries. These three plague pandemics originated in different parts of the world and spread along different paths. The devastation wrought by these pandemics not only affected nations and continents, but also led to profound social and economic changes throughout society.

THE PLAGUE OF JUSTINIAN

The Plague of Justinian, or Justinianic Plague, occurred in the sixth century and spanned the years 541–549 CE. It was named for Justinian, the Roman emperor in Constantinople, who contracted and recovered from the disease in 542 CE. This plague is believed to be the first and most well-known outbreak of the European epidemic of bubonic plague, which recurred for two centuries and had a death toll of an estimated twenty-five to one hundred million people, representing as much as half of Europe's population at the time of the first outbreak.

The Plague of Justinian, which spread throughout the Mediterranean Basin, Europe, and the Near East, started in Roman Egypt in 541 CE and then extended around the Mediterranean Sea through 544 CE. The epidemic lingered in Northern Europe and the Arabian Peninsula until 549 CE.

In 2013 researchers confirmed that the cause of the Plague of Justinian was *Yersinia pestis*, the same bacterium responsible for the Black Death, which ravaged Europe in the fourteenth century.

THE BLACK DEATH

The medieval pandemic originated in China in 1331, with plague eventually spreading along trade routes to Europe, North Africa, and the Middle East. The Black Death was the first major outbreak of the second great plague pandemic, which lasted from the fourteenth to the eighteenth centuries. This pandemic was referred to as the pestilence or pestilentia, with the term Black Death not being used until much later.

Between 1346 and 1353, the Black Death killed an estimated 75 to 200 million people in Eurasia and North Africa. Peaking between 1347 and 1351, the Black Death accounted for the deaths of at least a third of the population in Europe. A second major epidemic occurred in 1361, known as the *pestis secunda*, and accounted for the deaths of another 10 to 20 percent of Europe's population.

In the seventeenth century, pneumonic plague broke out in Europe. The Great Plague of London ravaged England from 1665 to 1666, killing around one hundred thousand people, or one fifth of London's population. The Great Fire of London in 1666, and the replacement of timber and thatch houses with brick and tile, contributed to a reduction in plague numbers and may have been a factor in ending the epidemic by disturbing the habitats of infected rats.

Smaller epidemics of this second great plague pandemic continued throughout the world into the eighteenth century, although none were as virulent as the Black Death.

THE THIRD PANDEMIC OF 1894

In 1855 the plague reemerged in Yunnan, a remote province of China. The disease then advanced along the tin and opium routes, spreading from capitals and provinces for decades until it reached Canton in 1894. From there it spread to Hong Kong and Bombay. By 1900 the plague had arrived in ports on every continent via infected rats traveling in steamships along international trade routes.

The third great plague pandemic continued to make itself known throughout the world for five more decades and didn't end until 1959. By that time more than fifteen million people had died, more than twelve million of them in India.

Question: Which infectious disease do historians believe killed Alexander the Great?

Answer: Alexander the Great (Alexander III of Macedon, 356–323 BCE) is a key figure in world history and is credited with the spread of Greek culture throughout the world. By the age of thirty, Alexander had created one of the largest empires of the ancient world through his extensive and unrelenting conquests.

Not surprisingly, Alexander made quite a few enemies during his brief life and, when he died at the age of thirty-two in the palace of Nebuchadnezzar II in Babylon, it was suspected that poisoning was the cause. However, some historians speculate that Alexander may have been felled by an infectious disease rather than nefarious revenge. Based on descriptions of Alexander's illness as chronicled in royal diaries, his symptoms were most consistent with typhoid fever or malaria, both of which were widespread in ancient Babylon.

Another theory about his death, based on an incident recorded by Plutarch, is that Alexander may have died of West Nile encephalitis. In Plutarch's account, when Alexander entered Babylon, he encountered a flock of ravens acting in a bizarre, uncharacteristic manner. This behavior could have been due to illness caused by West Nile virus and served to foreshadow Alexander's eventual demise.

Question: Which infectious diseases did George Washington survive?

Answer: Before he became father of a nation, George Washington battled a number of infectious diseases—including diphtheria, malaria, pneumonia, tuberculosis, and, most notably, smallpox. It was Washington's exposure to smallpox that led to a bold and risky move on his part: sanctioning the first state-funded mass inoculation program.

In 1751, at the age of nineteen, George Washington accompanied his half-brother Lawrence Washington to the island of Barbados. Lawrence had been plagued by tuberculosis and sought relief in the warmer island climate, which led to George contracting smallpox—a disease that had not yet made its way to his Virginia home. George, who was housebound for twenty-five days, wrote in his diary that he "was strongly attacked with the small Pox," but he was able to make a full recovery and return home.

Washington's exposure to smallpox would prove fortuitous years later, when the American Revolution brought soldiers carrying smallpox from England and Germany to his country. As a result, a smallpox epidemic quickly spread through the soldiers of the Continental Army. But because Washington had already survived smallpox, he had developed an immunity to the virus and was protected from the disease that ravaged his troops.

In 1777, Washington would go on to authorize the first mass military inoculation in history, with forty thousand soldiers being inoculated against smallpox. The outcome of the Revolutionary War was certainly altered by Washington's experience with smallpox and his determination to take aggressive measures to halt the spread of the disease among his soldiers.

Question: **Why and how were Native American populations in the United States affected by infectious diseases from Europe?**

Answer: By sampling ancient and modern mitochondrial DNA, which is passed down only from mothers to daughters, researchers have been able to calculate the demographic history of Native Americans. Based on their data, they estimate that the Native American population peaked around five thousand years ago and then dropped dramatically around five hundred years ago, just a few years after Christopher Columbus arrived in the New World.

Although these findings are not conclusive, extensive research indicates that the decline of indigenous populations can be traced to the introduction of new infectious diseases. In the years after Columbus arrived in 1492, Europeans brought many things from the Old World to the New World, including food crops, new populations—and highly contagious catastrophic illnesses.

The previously isolated Native American communities were suddenly exposed to infectious diseases to which they had no immunity. Researchers estimate that the influx of European settlers introduced or worsened at least thirty diseases in the New World, including these:

- Anthrax
- Botulism
- Bubonic plague
- Chicken pox
- Cholera
- Diphtheria
- Influenza
- Lyme disease
- Malaria
- Measles
- Scarlet fever
- Smallpox
- Syphilis
- Tetanus
- Toxoplasmosis
- Typhus
- Whooping cough
- Yellow fever

All told, the number of infections, illnesses, and deaths caused by Europeans introducing germs into the Americas was more devastating than the Black Death in medieval Europe. Researchers estimate that as much as 95 percent of the indigenous populations of the North American and South American continents died because of infectious diseases in just a few decades after Columbus first arrived.

Question: How was Fiji devastated by the introduction of measles?

Answer: The Republic of Fiji is an island country in the South Pacific Ocean, consisting of an archipelago of more than three hundred islands, more than one hundred of which are inhabited. Following intertribal wars in 1874, the Fiji islands hoped for a peaceful future under British colonialism. War gave way to a devastating infectious disease when Fijian chief Ratu Cakobau sailed to Australia in 1874 to ratify the Deed of Cession of the Fiji Islands to Queen Victoria. Unfortunately, Cakobau arrived in Sydney during an outbreak of measles.

Cakobau and some members of his traveling party caught the disease but received medical care in Sydney and were able to recover quickly from their illness. They returned to Fiji in January 1875, unaware that some members of the entourage were still infectious. The British authorities did not see a need for any of the travelers to quarantine after returning to Fiji, so the disease began to spread throughout the population within a week of their return home.

Distrustful of the British and believing the disease might have been deliberately visited on their country, many islanders refused to seek medical treatment. Instead, they opted for home remedies that did nothing to protect them from the highly contagious disease.

Within six months, one third of the population of Fiji—forty thousand people—had died as a result of the measles, making the Fiji measles epidemic the worst disaster in the small island nation's history.

Question: **Why is tuberculosis called the romantic disease?**

Answer: The term *tuberculosis* was coined by German physician Johann Lukas Schönlein in 1839. Nearly fifty years later, in March 1882, German physician and microbiologist Robert Koch announced the discovery of *Mycobacterium tuberculosis*, the bacteria that causes tuberculosis. At the time, tuberculosis was responsible for one out of every seven deaths in the United States and Europe.

Tuberculosis (or TB) has been called a number of names throughout history. It was *phthisis* in ancient Greece and *tabes* in ancient Rome. It was *schachepheth* in ancient Hebrew. In the eighteenth century, tuberculosis was called the white plague, due to the pale skin of those who were infected with it. In the nineteenth century, it was commonly referred to as consumption, a name that lingered even after it was officially named tuberculosis.

Although it's a disease that may have been around for as long as three million years, a surge of tuberculosis deaths in Western Europe during the eighteenth and nineteenth centuries coincided with the arrival of the Industrial Revolution—and Europe's Romantic era.

Romanticism was, in part, an impassioned response to the Industrial Revolution. It was an intellectual, artistic, literary, and musical movement that emphasized emotion over reason and glorified nature and history. The Romantic era was at its peak between the late-eighteenth century and the mid-nineteenth century, a time in which tuberculosis caused a large number of deaths and a high mortality rate among young and middle-aged adults.

When tuberculosis was running rampant in Europe, many writers and artists were being affected by the disease, either directly or through their families or loved ones. Their creative endeavors often reflected their experiences with the debilitating, and often deadly, consumption. As a result, the disease came to be associated with the Romantic movement. In fact, European women attempted to mimic the consumptive look of the disease by starving themselves and whitening their skin to achieve a highly desirable look of the era.

Beyond the physical attributes that became something of a fashion trend, contracting tuberculosis was believed to increase the emotional sensitivity of those afflicted with it. In time, suffering from tuberculosis became entwined with nineteenth-century ideals regarding beauty and creativity, lending those with the disease a mysterious and romantic air.

To die of consumption was a tragedy but—to the poets and their contemporaries, at least—it was a beautiful tragedy. After the death of his close friend John Keats, Percy Bysshe Shelley paid homage to him in *Adonais: An Elegy on the Death of John Keats*. Shelley did his part to contribute to the romanticism of consumption by styling Keats as a beautiful young god:

Peace, peace! He is not dead, he doth not sleep —
He hath awakened from the dream of life —

Keats was just twenty-five when he died of tuberculosis in 1831. The English Romantic poet was among the many celebrated writers, artists, and intellectuals whose lives and work were touched by tuberculosis. English writers Emily and Anne Brontë, and their brother, Branwell Brontë, all died of the disease within a few months of each other in 1848 and 1849. Their sister, writer Charlotte Brontë, also died of tuberculosis in 1855. English poet Elizabeth Barrett Browning died of tuberculosis in 1861, and Russian playwright Anton Chekhov succumbed to the disease in 1904. Their work, like the work of other creatives of the era, was infused with their experiences of living with, and dying from, tuberculosis.

Consumption had such a following during the era of Romanticism that Romantic poet George Gordon Byron, commonly known as Lord Byron, famously wrote, "How pale I look!—I should like, I think, to die of a consumption. Because then the women would all say, 'See that poor Byron—how interesting he looks in dying!'"

Alas, Lord Byron did not get his wish. After joining the fight for the Greek War of Independence in 1823, Byron died in 1824 at the age of thirty-six. His cause of death was a fever likely caused by sepsis—the body's serious and, in this case, deadly, response to an infection.

Question: What were tuberculosis sanatoriums, and do they still exist?

Answer: A sanatorium, also called a sanitarium or sanitorium, was a medical facility used for the treatment of long-term illness. In the late-nineteenth and early-twentieth centuries, sanatoriums were most often associated with the treatment of patients with tuberculosis.

Prior to the discovery of antibiotics in the 1940s, sanatoriums were intended to help tuberculosis patients fight off infection through a regimen of good nutrition and an abundance of rest. Fresh air, particularly in high altitudes and isolated areas, was also believed to be an important part of recovering from tuberculosis, and many sanatoriums were situated in mountainous areas of Europe and the United States.

Most sanatoriums were closed or converted to general hospitals within a few years after Albert Schatz's 1943 discovery of the tuberculosis-curing antibiotic streptomycin. Within a decade of the use of antibiotics, tuberculosis was no longer considered a major public health threat.

In the United States, Joseph Gleitsmann opened the first sanatorium in the picturesque mountains of Asheville, North Carolina, in 1875.

A. G. Holley State Hospital, which was opened in 1950 as the Southeast Florida State Sanatorium in Lantana, Florida, was the last tuberculosis sanatorium in the United States. It closed in July 2012.

CHAPTER 4

INFECTIOUS DISEASES IN THE ERA OF MODERN MEDICINE

How the Golden Age of Microbiology Changed the Way We Look at Disease

Question: When did our current understanding of infectious diseases begin?

Answer: It is the nature of humankind to seek explanations for the things we do not understand. Before the era of modern medicine, the causes of infectious disease were blamed on everything from bad air to angry gods to misaligned planets. Disease outbreaks have been the source of conspiracy theories and used as reasons to persecute entire ethnic groups.

Beliefs about microorganisms, the smallest forms of organic life, date back more than 2,500 years to ancient India in the fifth century BCE. Mahavira, a practitioner of the religious teaching of Jainism, hypothesized about the existence of tiny creatures, too small for the eye to see, which might live in the four major elements of the planet: air, earth, fire, and water. Mahavira's understanding of life was grounded in his religious beliefs, but he wasn't alone in thinking that life extended beyond what we can see—it just took several centuries to prove it.

It wasn't until the seventeenth century and the creation of a single-lens microscope that it became possible to prove the existence of microorganisms. Antonie van Leeuwenhoek (1632–1723), known as the father of microbiology, was a Dutch merchant-scientist whose work in microscopy, using microscopes of his own creation, contributed to the development of microbiology as a scientific discipline.

Microscopes opened up a whole new world to scientists and, as the quality of the lenses improved and their use became more prevalent, science began to identify and name what the microscopes revealed.

After steady scientific progress throughout the seventeenth and eighteenth centuries, the mid-nineteenth century brought an explosion of new theories and discoveries, rapidly advancing our understanding of infectious diseases. This period of intense progress, known as the Golden Age of Microbiology, spanned six decades, from 1850 until 1915. It is the foundation of our current understanding of the microorganisms that cause infectious diseases.

The field of microbiology is the basis for other scientific disciplines, including bacteriology, biochemistry, immunology, protozoology, and virology.

Question: What infectious disease was rumored to be caused by candy?

Answer: Kids love candy and, by the early twentieth century, candy shops were ubiquitous in every American city. So in 1916, when a terrifying new disease known as infantile paralysis began spreading throughout New York City and the Northeast United States, rumors began circulating that it might be related to children's voracious candy consumption.

Because the disease didn't follow the familiar paths of other known contagions and didn't discriminate on the basis of class—affecting the children of wealthy families as easily as the kids of impoverished communities—it was perhaps inevitable that a link would be suggested between the popularity of sweet treats and this new disease that was attacking so many families.

Infantile paralysis is known today as poliomyelitis or polio, and the link to candy consumption was eventually debunked. In time, researchers would come to understand poliomyelitis as an intestinal infection spread through fecal-oral transmission. Ironically, polio would go on to be virtually eradicated in the United States by 1979, thanks to two vaccines: Jonas Salk's injectable form, the inactivated polio vaccine (IPV) and Albert Sabin's oral polio vaccine (OPV)—a polio vaccine given to millions of children and adults throughout the 1960s...in a sugar cube.

Question: **When were medical face masks first used— and why?**

Answer: The use of face masks to prevent exposure to illness is not a modern concept. In fact, face masks—albeit unusual ones—have been in use for at least four centuries, even before the germ theory of disease took hold.

Seventeenth-century illustrations of plague doctors dressed in black coats, tall hats, and beak-like masks have come to symbolize the long period of European history when bubonic plague ravaged cities and villages unchecked. But the plague masks we have come to associate with the plague-doctor era were intended to protect the physician—not the patient—and were intended to shield the doctor from the miasma, or "bad air," that was believed to cause sickness.

The face mask used in health care today was a byproduct of the time when germ theory was developing and doctors began to consider how germs might infect open wounds. But wound protection began with the idea of killing the germs directly. In 1867, based on Louis Pasteur's description of germ-causing microscopic organisms, British surgeon Joseph Lister (1827–1912) introduced the use of antiseptics on wounds to eliminate germs. Although this method would eliminate germs at the surgical site, it did nothing to control the germs that might be introduced during surgery.

In 1897, German bacteriologist and hygienist Carl Flügge (1847–1923) published his findings on droplet infections, having noted that pathogens in respiratory droplets are responsible for disease transmission. The same year, he collaborated with Polish surgeon Johann von Mikulicz (1850–1905) on a paper that advocated the use of a facial covering—or a "mouth bandage"—during surgery.

Flügge and Mikulicz's advocacy contributed to the gradual introduction of face masks into surgical theaters in Europe. These simple masks were made of gauze and string tied so that the mask covered the nose, mouth, and beard. Thus began the gradual shift in focus from killing germs with chemicals to using a physical barrier to prevent the germs from spreading in the operating room. There remained considerable resistance to the use of face coverings in some medical circles, and surgical face masks were not used in the United States or Germany until the 1920s.

Despite being a controversial practice, health-care workers, as well as patients, slowly began adopting the practice of wearing face masks to protect from illness. Mandatory mask-wearing ordinances for medical workers, police personnel, and residents of several US cities (mostly in Western states) were issued during the 1918–19 influenza pandemic. A PSA put out by the Red Cross at the time relied on citizens' sense of wartime duty to promote a community obligation with the admonition, "The man or woman or child who will not wear a mask now is a dangerous slacker."

Face masks evolved as researchers tried to create the most effective germ-preventing covering to block the transmission of respiratory droplets both to and from the mask wearer. Early face coverings were made of porous gauze, first in a single layer and then in multiple layers, which would not have been capable of preventing all germ transmission. These masks gave way to washable masks made of multiple layers of cotton cloth, with metal parts that could be sterilized. These reusable masks were popular until the United States began experimenting with disposable single-use paper and fleece masks. By the mid-1960s, disposable masks were being used in operating rooms around the world.

Question: **Why is leprosy also called Hansen's disease?**

Answer: In 1873, Norwegian doctor Gerhard Henrik Armauer Hansen viewed the bacterium *Mycobaterium leprae* under a microscope and identified it as the causative agent of leprosy. In his honor, the disease is sometimes referred to as Hansen's disease.

Prior to Hansen's discovery that *M. leprae* was present in the tissues of all leprosy sufferers, the origins of leprosy were believed to be hereditary or miasmic in origin. Based on his epidemiological studies, Hansen became the first researcher to hypothesize that microorganisms could be the cause of human disease.

Question: **What is PPE?**

Answer: PPE stands for personal protective equipment and refers to protective clothing, helmets, face shields, face masks, goggles, gloves, respirators, and other equipment designed to protect the wearer from injury or exposure to infection or illness. Early PPE included cloth or rubber gloves and cloth masks, worn during surgery.

Today, PPE is commonly used in health-care facilities, such as hospitals, doctors' offices, and clinical labs, as well as other settings where the risk of germs could cause concern, such as veterinary hospitals and food production and preparation facilities. Properly used, PPE works as a physical barrier between the wearer's skin, mouth, nose, and eyes and the pathogens, or germs, that cause viral and bacterial infections. This barrier serves to block the transmission of germs in blood, body fluids, or respiratory secretions.

The US Food and Drug Administration (FDA) regulates the use of PPE in the United States, including medical gowns, gloves, N95 respirators, and surgical masks. All PPE that is intended for medical use must follow the FDA's regulations and meet certain standards for protection.

Question: What are the different types of face masks, and how can they protect me from becoming infected with COVID-19?

Answer: The COVID-19 pandemic has raised public awareness about the use of personal protective equipment (PPE) in general and face masks in particular. There are many types of commercially available face masks, and they have varying degrees of effectiveness. To be reasonably assured that you get the proper protection, it is important to select the appropriate face mask.

N95 RESPIRATORS

N95 respirators are designed to create a tight, fitted seal around the nose and mouth. Worn correctly, an N95 respirator can block at least 95 percent of small airborne particles (hence their name). N95s are made of many layers of fine polypropylene fibers, which use static electricity to trap incoming and outgoing particles and droplets.

SURGICAL MASKS

Surgical masks are disposable coverings that are most often made of paper but can also be made of polypropylene. Unlike N95 respirators, surgical masks are primarily intended to protect other people from the wearer. To this end, they work to block large-particle droplets or splashes in the air. Although surgical masks can block the majority of respiratory droplets emitted by an infected person, the protection from smaller particles can vary widely, from 30 to 80 percent, depending on the mask.

FABRIC MASKS

Fabric masks can be made of a variety of materials, but most are made of cotton or a cotton-blend fabric. Research suggests that the most effective fabric masks have two layers of a tight-weave fabric with a built-in pocket for a disposable or washable filter. A filter made of polypropylene, the same material found in N95 respirators, offers the best protection for the wearer. A two-layer tight-weave cotton mask without a filter can block about 35 percent of small particles, and the addition of a polypropylene filter can add another 35 percent of additional protection.

Question: **What does MMR stand for in the MMR vaccine?**

Answer: The initials in the MMR vaccine stand for measles, mumps, and rubella. To protect against these diseases, the CDC recommends that children receive two doses of the MMR vaccine, with the first dose at twelve to fifteen months of age, and the second dose at four to six years of age. Adults and teens who did not receive the MMR vaccine as children can also receive the vaccine.

There is also an MMRV vaccine, with the *V* standing for varicella, or chicken pox. This vaccine is licensed for use in children from twelve months to twelve years of age.

Question: **What is the 80/20 rule?**

Answer: Epidemiologists use the 80/20 rule, also known as the Pareto principle or Pareto rule, to explain how asymptomatic carriers can spread an infectious disease throughout a population

The Pareto principle wasn't originally intended as a medical term, but rather was borrowed from the world of business and economics. As the story goes, Italian sociologist, political scientist, and economist Vilfredo Federico Damaso Pareto (1848–1923) was inspired by his vegetable garden to formulate the 80/20 rule when he saw that 20 percent of his plants produced as much as 80 percent of his vegetable crop. Pareto applied his analysis to the distribution of wealth in Italy and noted that, in business and industry, 80 percent of production is generated by just 20 percent of companies.

Distilled to simplicity, the Pareto principle assumes that 80 percent of the results of an activity will come from only 20 percent of the actions required to achieve the results. The Pareto principle, or 80/20 rule, has been applied to all areas of life, from the natural world to the business world to medicine.

The Pareto principle is used as a rule of thumb by epidemiologists in speculating that 80 percent of infectious disease transmission is conducted by only 20 percent of the population—many of whom are asymptomatic carriers of the disease.

Question: What is a super spreader?

Answer: A super spreader is a highly contagious person who is able to transmit an infectious disease to many other people. Super spreaders are often asymptomatic and may transmit the disease without knowing it.

According to the 80/20 rule, or Pareto principle, 80 percent of disease transmission is caused by just 20 percent of the population, the super spreaders. Whether a person becomes a super spreader is based on a combination of factors, including the characteristics of the disease as well as the person's own biology, behavior, and environment. Because super spreaders are often asymptomatic, their lack of symptoms can allow them to transmit the disease to many people without even being aware that they're sick.

Super spreading can happen with any infectious disease. The most notorious super spreader in history was most likely Mary Mallon, who got the nickname Typhoid Mary for her prolific and asymptomatic spread of typhoid, but researchers have identified super spreaders in outbreaks of several infectious diseases, including tuberculosis, measles, SARS (severe acute respiratory syndrome) and MERS (Middle East respiratory syndrome), and Ebola.

Question: **What vaccines do we have now to protect us from the diseases our grandparents may have experienced when they were kids?**

Answer: Depending on how old you are, your grandparents and parents likely experienced the threat of a number of infectious diseases when they were children before there were safe and effective vaccines available to protect against them.

Here is a list of vaccines and when they were first licensed in the United States:

- *1914*: Rabies and typhoid
- *1915*: Pertussis
- *1923*: Diphtheria
- *1935*: Yellow fever
- *1937*: Tetanus
- *1945*: Influenza A and influenza B
- *1947*: Combination tetanus and diphtheria (Td)
- *1949*: Combination diphtheria, tetanus, and pertussis (DTaP)
- *1955*: Polio (Salk, inactivated poliovirus vaccine)
- *1963*: Measles
- *1967*: Mumps
- *1969*: Rubella
- *1971*: Combination measles, mumps, and rubella (MMR)

In the United States, the immunization schedules for children and adults are updated annually by the Centers for Disease Control and Prevention, the American Academy of Pediatrics, and the American Academy of Family Physicians to accommodate new recommendations and changes to existing recommendations. Current recommended vaccines for children from birth to age 18 include the following:

- Diphtheria, tetanus, and pertussis (in combination as the DTaP vaccine)
- Hepatitis A
- Hepatitis B
- Hib (Haemophilus influenzae type b)
- Human papillomavirus (HPV)
- Influenza (Flu)
- Measles, mumps, and rubella (in combination as the MMR vaccine)
- Meningococcal

- Polio (inactivated poliovirus, IPV)
- Pneumococcal
- Rotavirus
- Varicella (chicken pox)

Question: **What is the difference between a bacterial infection and a viral infection?**

Answer: For most of us, the important difference between a bacterial infection and a viral infection is that antibiotics can be used to treat a bacterial infection but are ineffective against a viral infection. Unfortunately, the misuse of antibiotics has led to a number of bacterial infectious diseases that are resistant to antibiotic treatment (often referred to as drug-resistant).

BACTERIAL INFECTIONS

Bacterial infections are caused by single-celled microorganisms called bacteria. These microorganisms can be found just about everywhere, including in soil, in water, and in and on the human body. Many types can survive in extreme temperatures. Most bacteria are harmless but some types cause infection and illness.

These are some examples of diseases caused by bacteria:

- Anthrax
- Bacterial foodborne illness (caused by E. coli, Salmonella, or Shigella)
- Bacterial meningitis
- Bacterial skin infections (such as MRSA)
- Bacterial urinary tract infections
- Botulism
- Chlamydia
- Cholera
- Gonorrhea
- Lyme disease

- Pertussis (whooping cough)
- Pneumococcal pneumonia
- Strep throat
- Syphilis
- Tetanus
- Tuberculosis

In the treatment of bacterial infections, antibiotics work to either kill the bacteria or to prevent it from growing and multiplying.

VIRAL INFECTIONS

Viral infections are caused by infectious microorganisms made up of a piece of genetic material surrounded by a protein shell. Viruses are even smaller than bacteria and are parasitic—to survive, they require a living host. A virus takes over a host cell inside a person, animal, or plant, which is where it lives out its life cycle. Once inside the host cell, it is able to use the cellular material to reproduce and then release new viruses from the host cell, a process that sometimes kills the host cell.

Some examples of diseases caused by viruses include the following:

- Chicken pox
- Common cold
- Ebola
- Herpes simplex virus (HSV)
- HIV/AIDs
- Human papillomavirus (HPV)
- Infectious mononucleosis (mono)
- Influenza
- Measles
- Norovirus
- Polio
- Rabies
- Rubella

- Viral hepatitis (A, B, C, D, and E)
- Viral meningitis
- West Nile virus

Although antibiotics are ineffective against viruses, there are antiviral drugs that can help fight some viral infections, such as hepatitis B and C, herpes, HIV/AIDS, and influenza. The course of treatment for many viral infections is to provide relief for the symptoms while the immune system does its job clearing the infection from the body.

Question: What is the CDC—and what do they do?

Answer: Headquartered in Atlanta, Georgia, the Centers for Disease Control and Prevention (CDC) is a US public health institute. Operating as a federal agency under the Department of Health and Human Services, the mission of the CDC is to increase the health security of the United States by protecting the nation from health, safety, and security threats, both foreign and domestic.

The CDC opened on July 1, 1946, as the Communicable Disease Center, with fewer than four hundred employees and a budget of ten million dollars. At the time, its main goal was to prevent malaria from spreading across the country. Under the leadership of its founder, US physician Joseph Mountin (1891–1952), the CDC expanded its mission to include a focus on disease surveillance.

In 1992, the United States Congress enacted the CDC's name change to the Centers for Disease Control and Prevention, reflecting the evolution of the CDC's mission since its humble beginnings fighting malaria, and honoring the importance of the center's role in the prevention of disease, injury, and disability.

Today, the CDC is a vast organization of centers, institutes, and offices (CIOs), employing around eleven thousand staff members and working with an annual budget of almost twelve billion dollars.

Question: How does the World Health Organization look out for the global population?

Answer: The World Health Organization (WHO) is headquartered in Geneva, Switzerland, with six semi-autonomous branches in other regions. The WHO is a specialized agency of the United Nations, serving as the coordinating authority on issues of international health. Countries that are members of the United Nations may become members of the WHO by accepting the agency's constitution. Other countries can be admitted under different terms. Currently, there are 194 member states in the WHO.

Established in 1948, the WHO's mission is to "promote health, keep the world safe, and serve the vulnerable." Among the WHO's goals include coordinating responses to public health emergencies, promoting human health and well-being, and advocating for universal healthcare.

The World Health Assembly (WHA) is the decision-making body of the WHO and is made up of representatives of the member states. The WHA meets annually in May to discuss health policies, set priorities, and approve the WHO's budget and goals. The *World Health Report* is the WHO's annual report, assessing global health issues and health statistics.

The WHO has served in a leadership role for several world health achievements, including the eradication of smallpox.

The WHO has a biennial budget of more than four billion dollars, which comes from the assessed contributions of member-state governments and voluntary contributions from member states, private organizations, and individuals.

Question: What is the National Institutes of Health?

Answer: The National Institutes of Health (NIH) is the largest biomedical research agency in the world and operates under the United States Department of Health and Human Services. Headquartered in Bethesda, Maryland, the NIH began as the Hygienic Laboratory in 1887 and today is made up of twenty-seven centers and institutes focused on different biomedical disciplines.

The NIH guides the behavioral and medical health research in the nation. Among the goals of the agency are to advance the protection and improvement of the nation's health. The NIH has been the leader in research for a number of scientific advances, including vaccines for hepatitis, Hib, and HPV.

Question: What is the Food and Drug Administration?

Answer: The Food and Drug Administration (FDA) is another US federal agency that operates under the Department of Health and Human Services. Founded in 1906 and headquartered in Silver Spring, Maryland, the

FDA is a regulatory agency responsible for protecting and promoting public health.

The FDA controls and monitors food safety, prescription and over-the-counter medications, vaccines, pet foods and animal feed, medical and veterinary devices, and other products as they relate to public health and safety.

Question: **What is the difference between eradicating a disease and eliminating a disease?**

Answer: A disease is eradicated when deliberate efforts lead to the permanent global reduction of that disease to zero incidences of infection caused by a specific agent. When a disease has been eradicated, the intervention measures previously used are no longer required because the agent that caused the disease is no longer present.

A disease is eliminated when deliberate efforts lead to a reduction to zero incidences of infection caused by a specific agent in a defined geographic area. A disease can be eliminated from a geographic region without being eradicated globally, but strategies remain necessary to prevent the disease from reemerging or spreading after it has been eliminated from a specific region.

So far the World Health Organization recognizes only two diseases as having been eradicated worldwide:

- Smallpox, which is caused by the variola virus, was eradicated in 1980.

- Rinderpest, which is caused by the rinderpest virus, was eradicated in 2011.

Smallpox was an ancient disease that caused devastating epidemics throughout history. Rinderpest was a bovine disease that caused the deaths of cattle herds throughout Europe and Africa from the eighteenth century to the twentieth century.

To determine whether a disease can be eradicated, certain scientific, political, and economic criteria must be considered. Both smallpox and rinderpest had certain characteristics that made their eradication possible. When scientists study the potential for eradicating infectious diseases, two conditions must be met:

- The disease must be an infectious disease. Noninfectious diseases, such as cancer or heart disease, cannot be eradicated.

- The measures necessary to fight the disease must exist. As science develops, this condition can, and does, change.

Certain characteristics of a disease make it more likely that eradication is possible. They are as follows:

- The disease has only one host.
- The disease is caused by a small number of pathogens.
- The disease is recognizable and diagnosable.
- The disease has already been eliminated from at least one geographic area.
- The disease burden is considered high, and there is financial, political, and community support for its eradication.

In addition to the eradication of smallpox and rinderpest, several other diseases have been targeted by the WHO for global eradication, including the following:

- Guinea worm disease
- Lymphatic filariasis
- Measles
- Mumps
- Polio
- Rubella
- Yaws

Due in large part to widespread national vaccination efforts, several infectious diseases have already been eliminated in the United States, including these:

- Bovine babesiosis (Texas cattle fever, which effects cattle and wildlife)
- Diphtheria
- Malaria
- Measles
- Polio
- Rubella
- Smallpox
- Yellow fever

Question: What is mad cow disease? Can a person get it by eating beef?

Answer: Bovine spongiform encephalopathy (BSE) is the scientific name of the disease more commonly known as mad cow disease. This neurodegenerative disease is caused by abnormalities in a protein found on cell surfaces. This protein, called a prion, becomes altered and acts as an infectious agent that attacks and destroys the central nervous system—the brain and the spinal cord—of the animal.

BSE was first identified in the United Kingdom in 1986, but researchers believe it may have been around for a decade or more before its discovery. The disease has a long incubation period, so it can take several years from the time a cow is infected with BSE until the onset of physical symptoms. These symptoms include trouble walking, abnormal ("mad") behavior, and weight loss. Once symptoms appear, death follows in a matter of weeks or months.

BSE cannot be transmitted to humans either by live cows or by beef. However, it is believed that infected cows can transmit a form of the disease to humans called variant Creutzfeldt-Jakob disease (vCJD), a rapidly progressive brain disorder with dementia-like symptoms that is always fatal. Cooking, which can kill disease-causing organisms in food, does not affect prions. Therefore, a person could become infected with vCJD by eating beef products that contain central nervous tissue—the brain or spinal cord—from an infected animal.

Question: What's the difference between chicken pox and shingles? And if you've had chicken pox, are you more likely to get shingles?

Answer: Both chicken pox and shingles are caused by the varicella-zoster virus, but they are not the same illness.

Chicken pox is a primary varicella infection that most often affects children and usually has mild symptoms. A person who has had a primary varicella infection usually has immunity against chicken pox for life. However, the varicella-zoster virus remains latent in the person's body.

Herpes zoster (shingles) is caused by the reactivation of the varicella-zoster virus in the body. Shingles most often affects older people, but young adults and children can also get it. The pain that accompanies a shingles infection can be severe and last for a long time after the shingles rash has faded. A person who has a compromised or suppressed immune system, which could be caused by, among other factors, cancer, HIV, an organ transplant, or immunosuppressive medications, is at increased risk for herpes zoster.

The first vaccine to protect against varicella was licensed in the United States in 1995. In 2006, the first vaccine against herpes zoster was licensed. The chicken pox vaccine is recommended for children and adults who have never had chicken pox or been vaccinated against it. The CDC recommends that children receive the first of two doses at age twelve to fifteen months and the second dose at age four to six years. It recommends that healthy adults older than fifty receive two doses of the shingles vaccine, two to six months apart.

A person who has experienced a natural chicken pox infection can develop shingles. Children who have gotten the varicella vaccine can also develop shingles, but the vaccine helps reduce their risk.

In the United States, around one million people get shingles each year and one out of three people will develop shingles in their lifetime. The best way to be protected from shingles is to be vaccinated. The vaccine may not prevent the shingles virus, but it can reduce the risk of long-lasting pain.

CHAPTER 5

EVERYTHING WE KNOW ABOUT INFLUENZA

*History of the Flu—And Why
You Should Get a Flu Shot*

Question: Why was the strain of influenza that caused the 1918 pandemic called the Spanish flu?

Answer: In the spring of 1918, the deadliest strain of influenza in modern history began making its way around the world, infecting as much as 40 percent of the world's population over the next eighteen months. In time it would become known as the 1918 flu pandemic, but in the fall of 1918, it was commonly called the Spanish flu or the Spanish Lady in the United States and Europe.

Despite its name, it's unlikely that the Spanish flu originated in Spain. World War I was winding down when the flu first took hold, and Spain was one of a few European countries that had remained neutral during the war. Although wartime censors in the nations of the Allied and Central powers were keen on suppressing the news of the flu to avoid damaging their citizens' morale, the Spanish media had no such concerns and reported on the flu's toll.

News of this deadly influenza strain soon spread nearly as quickly as the flu itself, especially after Spain's King Alfonso XIII fell ill. Countries that had been under a media blackout believed the influenza strain must have originated in Spain, while Spanish citizens thought the flu had come from France and began calling it the French flu.

Researchers still aren't sure where the 1918 influenza strain originated. Because World War I was going on at the same time, it's believed that the war contributed to the virus spreading more quickly around the world than it would have otherwise. Britain, China, and France were possible nations of origin, as was the United States, where the first known case of the deadly strain was reported at a Kansas military base in March 1918.

Question: Did scientists reconstruct the virus that caused the 1918 influenza pandemic?

Answer: The 1918 influenza pandemic lasted for two years and ravaged entire nations. The United States suffered 675,000 deaths. Worldwide, the pandemic killed 20 to 50 million people.

Understanding why that particular strain of influenza was so deadly is a key component to helping scientists, researchers, and public health officials understand and prepare for future influenza pandemics.

In 2005, scientists at the Centers for Disease Control and Prevention (CDC) were able to reconstruct the 1918 influenza strain. This allowed researchers to identify the specific genes that made the 1918 flu so deadly. This knowledge will help researchers develop new influenza vaccines and treatments, which could save lives should the world ever face a similar pandemic.

Question: How did the 1918 influenza pandemic affect life expectancy?

Answer: Although it's the death toll—twenty to fifty million people worldwide—that is most often the focus of any discussion of the 1918 influenza pandemic, one interesting bit of information would seem to be more dramatic than it really was: the pandemic altered the life expectancy of the population.

In 1918, when the flu began spreading from one population to the next, scientists hadn't yet discovered flu viruses. But we now know that the 1918 pandemic was caused by an influenza A (H1N1) virus. Worldwide, as many as five hundred million people were infected by the virus, with the flu spreading quickly throughout communities in what researchers now believe were three distinct waves. The first wave of the flu virus occurred in the spring of 1918, the second in the fall of 1918, and the third and final wave in the winter and spring of 1919.

When it comes to calculating life expectancy, actuaries use a summary indicator called period life expectancy (PLE), which reflects the health of a population at a particular time. The life expectancy of a person at birth is based on a snapshot of the population's mortality at a given time. In just one year, from 1917 to 1918, the 1918 pandemic reduced the PLE in the United States for both males and females by 11.8 years.

But despite the impact of the pandemic on the United States—which lasted from 1918 until 1920 and infected more than 25 percent of the population—there was no lasting effect on PLE. In fact, the estimates increased for both sexes in 1919 and were higher than they had been in 1917.

Question: **When was the first flu vaccine created?**

Answer: In the wake of the tremendous loss of life caused by the 1918 influenza pandemic, researchers were committed to developing a flu vaccine. But several more decades would pass before a vaccine became widely available.

In the 1930s, researchers were able to isolate influenza viruses from people and prove that influenza was caused by a virus and not a bacterium. Thomas Francis Jr., an American virologist and epidemiologist, was the first person in the United States to isolate the influenza virus. He discovered two strains of influenza. Once these different virus strains—known as influenza A and influenza B —were identified, work began on an inactivated flu vaccine. The first clinical trials of influenza vaccine were conducted in the mid-1930s.

With the support of the US Army, Francis and Jonas Salk—the latter would go on to develop a polio vaccine in 1952—developed an influenza vaccine that was distributed to military troops during World War II. Their use of fertilized chicken eggs to develop the vaccine is a procedure that is still in use to produce most flu vaccines today.

The original influenza vaccine included only an inactivated influenza A virus. In 1942, a bivalent (two-component) vaccine was created, which offered protection against both influenza A and influenza B viruses. In 1945, the inactivated influenza vaccine was licensed for civilian use.

Question: How many different types of influenza virus are there?

Answer: There are four known types of influenza viruses: A, B, C, and D.

- Influenza A and B viruses cause human seasonal epidemics of disease.
- Influenza A viruses are the only viruses known to cause flu pandemics.

- Influenza A viruses are divided into subtypes based on proteins on the surface of the virus.
- The two proteins on the surface of influenza A viruses are hemagglutinin (H) and neuraminidase (N).
- There are 18 hemagglutinin subtypes (H1–H18) and 11 neuraminidase subtypes (N1–N11).
- There are potentially 198 subtypes of influenza A, but only 131 subtypes have been detected in nature.
- Influenza C viruses cause mild illness and aren't believed to cause human flu epidemics.
- Influenza D viruses affect primarily cattle and aren't known to infect people.

Question: **How are different influenza viruses named?**

Answer: In the United States, the Centers for Disease Control and Prevention (CDC) follows the internationally accepted naming convention.

These are the steps followed in naming an influenza virus:

- The virus type: A, B, C, or D.
- The host of origin: swine, equine, chicken, and so on. For human-origin viruses, no host of origin designation is given.
- The geographic origin of the virus.
- The strain number of the virus.
- The year of collection.

For influenza A viruses, the hemagglutinin and neuraminidase antigen descriptions are given in parentheses, for example, influenza A(H1N1) virus or influenza A(H5N1) virus.

The 2009–10 pandemic influenza virus was given the name influenza A(H1N1)pdm09 to distinguish it from the seasonal influenza A(H1N1) in the same year.

An influenza virus that usually circulates in swine but has begun infecting humans is called a variant virus and is designated with the letter *v*; for example, influenza A(H3N2)v virus.

Question: **Who should get a flu vaccine, and how many people get the vaccine each year?**

Answer: Most people who get the flu will experience a mild illness that lasts less than two weeks and does not require the care of a physician or antiviral drugs. However, some populations are at higher risk of developing complications if they get the flu, including the following:

- Adults older than sixty-five
- Children younger than five, especially those younger than two
- People who have chronic illnesses, such as asthma, diabetes, or heart, kidney, or liver disease
- People with a weakened immune system
- People with a body mass index (BMI) of 40 or greater
- Pregnant women and women up to two weeks postpartum
- Residents of long-term care facilities and nursing homes

The CDC recommends that everyone older than six months receive an annual flu vaccine, which is available as an injection or a nasal spray. The vaccine's effectiveness varies from season to season, and even among age groups and vaccine types. But studies show that the flu vaccine still reduces the risk of flu illness by 40 to 60 percent for the overall population in seasons when the flu vaccine is well matched to the viruses in circulation.

Flu vaccination coverage in the United States varies from year to year and from age group to age group. During the 2018–19 flu season, the flu vaccine rate among children six months to seventeen years was 62.6 percent, a 4.7 percent increase from the 2017–18 flu season. The flu vaccine rate for people eighteen years and older was 45.3 percent, an 8.2 percent increase from the previous flu season.

Question: Why does the flu vaccine have to be redesigned every year?

Answer: New influenza vaccines are developed each year to keep up with the constantly changing flu viruses. More than one hundred influenza centers around the world conduct year-round studies on influenza to determine which vaccine viruses will be used to create new seasonal influenza vaccines.

The seasonal influenza vaccines are designed to protect against the flu viruses that researchers believe are most likely to be circulating in a given season. Trivalent (three-component) and quadrivalent (four-component) influenza vaccines are currently available, which means a single vaccine includes protection against three or four of the flu viruses circulating in a particular year. The flu shot includes only influenza A and B viruses and does not protect against influenza C or D viruses, because influenza C viruses are considered to cause only mild illness and influenza D viruses are not known to cause illness in humans.

Every year, new seasonal influenza vaccines are developed using one influenza A(H1N1) virus, one influenza A(H3N2) virus, and one or two influenza B viruses, depending on whether a trivalent or a quadrivalent vaccine is being developed.

Question: **Which flu viruses have caused pandemics?**

Answer: An influenza pandemic is caused by a new (novel) influenza A virus, one that is different from current and recent human seasonal influenza A viruses.

There are two ways influenza viruses can change and a new influenza virus can emerge: through antigenic drift and through antigenic shift.

Antigenic drift is a small change (or mutation) in the genes of an influenza virus that leads to changes in the surface proteins of the virus. The small changes can produce viruses that the body's immune system doesn't recognize, which makes a person susceptible to flu infection again even if they've already had the flu. Because influenza viruses are changing all the time due to antigenic drift, the flu vaccine must be updated as often as every year to keep up with the changes.

Antigenic shift is a sudden, major change in an influenza A virus that results in new proteins in influenza viruses that infect humans. This shift can happen when an influenza virus from an animal population becomes able to infect humans. Influenza A viruses are hosted by different animals, including birds and pigs, and are constantly changing. Rarely, one of these nonhuman flu viruses will change in a way that makes it possible for people to be infected and for the new influenza A virus to be spread through person-to-person contact.

Influenza A viruses undergo both antigenic drift and antigenic shift, and are the only influenza viruses known to cause pandemics. Influenza B viruses change only through antigenic drift.

There have been four influenza pandemics since the beginning of the twentieth century:

- *1918 pandemic, H1N1 virus*: Although there is no consensus on where this influenza virus originated, it was first reported by Spain and was called the Spanish flu. Caused by an H1N1 virus with genes of avian origin, this influenza A virus caused an estimated 20 to 50 million deaths worldwide and around 675,000 deaths in the United States.

- *1957–58 pandemic, H2N2 virus*: Emerging in East Asia, this influenza virus was also known as the Asian flu and originated from an avian influenza A virus. This influenza pandemic caused an estimated 1.1 million deaths worldwide and 116,000 deaths in the United States.

- *1968–69 pandemic, the H3N2 virus*: Known as the Hong Kong flu because that was the location of the first reported outbreak, this influenza A virus contained two genes from an avian influenza A virus as well as an enzyme from the 1957 H2N2 virus. There were an estimated 1 million deaths worldwide and about 100,000 deaths in the United States. The H3N2 virus continues to circulate worldwide as a seasonal influenza A virus.

- **2009–10 H1N1 pandemic, the (H1N1)pdm09 virus**: The influenza A virus that caused the 2009 pandemic was referred to as the swine flu. The 2009 H1N1 influenza was called a quadruple genetic reassortment virus by scientists because individual gene segments of the virus originated from humans, birds, North American pigs, and Eurasian pigs. During the pandemic, an estimated 284,000 people died worldwide, with 12,469 deaths in the United States. The (H1N1)pdm09 virus continues to circulate as a seasonal influenza virus.

Question: **Can you get the flu from the flu shot?**

Answer: It is a myth that getting the flu vaccine can cause the flu. There are a variety of reasons someone might experience flu-like symptoms even if he or she gets the flu shot, but the vaccine itself does not cause flu illness.

The flu shot contains either inactivated viruses or only a single protein from the flu virus, while the nasal spray vaccine contains live viruses that are too weak to cause illness. But there are several reasons someone might feel sick after getting a flu vaccine, including the following:

- **A reaction to the vaccine**: Some people experience mild symptoms, including muscle aches and fever, after receiving a flu vaccine. This is likely a side effect of the body producing protective antibodies.

- **The flu shot hasn't had a chance to start working**: It can take around two weeks for the flu vaccine to be fully effective. If a person is exposed to the flu virus either before or during that time, that individual could catch the flu.

- **The flu vaccine doesn't match the flu viruses in circulation**: The effectiveness of the flu vaccine depends, in part, on how well it is matched to the viruses that are circulating that season. If the vaccine isn't a good match for the viruses a person is exposed to, he or she could get the flu—but the vaccine will still offer some protection, lessening the severity of the illness and reducing the risk of complications.

- **Other illnesses**: Many illnesses can have flu-like symptoms, including the common cold. The only way to be sure an illness is the flu is to be tested.

Question: Is the stomach flu really the flu?

Answer: Remember that influenza is a respiratory disease. What people may call the stomach flu—with symptoms including diarrhea, nausea, and vomiting—rarely has anything to do with influenza. Although these symptoms might be present if someone has the flu, they are more common in children than adults and are not the main symptoms of the flu.

Viral gastroenteritis, also called stomach flu, is an inflammation of the stomach and intestines that can be caused by several different viruses—but it is not related to influenza. It is highly contagious and can be spread through close contact with people who are infected or through contaminated food or water.

Several viruses can cause viral gastroenteritis. Two of the most common are norovirus and rotavirus.

Norovirus is the most common cause of foodborne illness and is more often found in crowded spaces. It can affect both children and adults, with symptoms lasting from one to three days. Norovirus is the leading cause of gastroenteritis worldwide. Although it can occur at any time of the year, most outbreaks in the United States occur between November and April. Symptoms include the following:

- Body aches
- Diarrhea
- Fever
- Nausea

Rotavirus most commonly affects infants and young children, although asymptomatic adults can spread it. Symptoms can last from three to eight days and can occur at any time of the year, although peak times in the United States are in the winter and spring. Symptoms include the following:

- Diarrhea
- Loss of appetite
- Vomiting

Other illnesses that can mimic the symptoms of viral gastroenteritis, or "stomach flu," include these:

- Digestive disorders, such as celiac disease, Crohn's disease, or ulcerative colitis
- Food intolerances, such as lactose intolerance
- Medications, such as antibiotics or antacids with magnesium

Finally, "stomach flu" symptoms of an intestinal infection could also be caused by bacteria, such as *E. coli* or *Salmonella*, or by a parasite, such as *Giardia*.

Question: **How serious is the flu in any given year? How many people die of the flu each year?**

Answer: The World Health Organization estimates that 290,000 to 650,000 people worldwide die as a result of the flu each year. In the United States, the CDC estimates that 12,000 to 61,000 people have died each year since 2010 as a result of the flu.

The annual number of deaths varies based on several factors, including which influenza virus strains are circulating in a given season, how well that season's vaccine works against those strains, and how many people get the flu vaccine.

The CDC measures the annual disease burden of influenza in the United States—that is, the estimated numbers of illnesses, medical visits, hospitalizations, and deaths—as well as the impact the influenza vaccine has on these numbers.

Based on preliminary burden estimates for the 2019–20 flu season (from October 1, 2019, to April 4, 2020), the CDC has these estimates:

- 39 to 56 million flu illnesses
- 18 to 26 million flu medical visits
- 410,000 to 740,000 flu hospitalizations
- 24,000 to 62,000 flu deaths

Influenza surveillance in the United States does not reflect all of the flu cases in a given flu season, so the CDC provides estimated ranges to better indicate the larger burden of influenza.

Question: **What is the difference between the flu and the common cold?**

Answer: Influenza and the common cold are both upper-respiratory illnesses that can have similar symptoms, but they're caused by different viruses. It can be difficult to determine, based on symptoms alone, whether someone has the flu or a cold, but cold symptoms are generally milder than flu symptoms, and a cold, unlike the flu, usually does not lead to more serious illnesses.

The onset of flu symptoms is usually sudden, and they can be severe and last for one to two weeks. Symptoms of the flu can include the following:

- Body aches (usual and often severe)
- Chills (common)
- Cough and chest discomfort (common)
- Fatigue (usual)

- Fever (usual, lasts three to four days)
- Headache (common)
- Sneezing, stuffy nose (sometimes)
- Sore throat (sometimes)
- Vomiting and diarrhea (sometimes, but it's more common in children than adults)

In contrast, the onset of cold symptoms is usually gradual, and symptoms usually improve in seven to ten days (although they can linger for as long as two weeks). Fever and headache rarely accompany a cold and, although other symptoms of flu may present, they are usually milder when the illness is a cold. A runny or stuffy nose is a frequent cold symptom but is less common with the flu.

Rhinovirus is the most common cold-causing virus and is responsible for as much as 75 percent of colds in adults. It's also highly contagious. Unfortunately, there may never be a vaccine for the common cold because there are more than 160 different strains of rhinovirus.

Question: **Why is there a "flu season," and does that mean you can't catch the flu at other times of the year?**

Answer: Influenza is an airborne infectious respiratory disease. Cases tend to peak during colder temperatures. The flu virus is more likely to be transmitted from person to person in cold weather because the virus has a protective gel-like coating, which allows it to survive in the air. The coating degrades in warm temperatures, making transmission more difficult and reducing the rate of infection.

In the northern hemisphere, flu season usually begins in October and peaks between December and February, but flu cases can continue until as late as May. In the southern hemisphere, flu season is from April to September.

So although flu activity is more prevalent in the colder months, you can still get the flu at any time of the year.

CHAPTER 6

SEXUALLY TRANSMITTED DISEASES AND THE HIV/AIDS EPIDEMIC

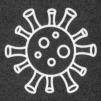

*How the "Modern Plague"
Changed Our View of
Disease and Sex*

Question: What's the difference between an STI (sexually transmitted infection) and an STD (sexually transmitted disease)?

Answer: Generally speaking, the terms *STI* and *STD* are interchangeable—but sometimes *STI* is a more accurate and preferred description for the group of infections transmitted through sexual contact.

Sexually transmitted infections can be asymptomatic or cause only mild symptoms, making detection more difficult. For those infections that can cause disease, not every infection will develop into a disease. For example, most women who become infected with HPV (human papilloma virus) will not develop cervical cancer, the disease that can be caused by HPV.

Sexually transmitted infections and diseases can be caused by bacteria, viruses, or parasites. Bacterial and parasitic infections can be treated and cured with antibiotics. STIs caused by viruses can be treated to relieve the symptoms but cannot be cured. Some common sexually transmitted infections include the following:

- Bacterial vaginosis
- Chlamydia
- Gonorrhea
- Hepatitis
- Herpes
- HIV/AIDS
- Human papillomavirus (HPV) infection

- Pelvic inflammatory disease (PID)
- Syphilis
- Trichomoniasis

Question: How common are sexually transmitted infections?

Answer: Sexually transmitted infections (STIs) are very common. According to the World Health Organization, more than one million STIs are acquired worldwide *every day*.

STIs have a substantial effect on reproductive and sexual health. More than thirty different types of bacteria, viruses, and parasites can be transmitted through sexual contact, including vaginal, anal, and oral sex. These eight STIs are responsible for the most transmissions:

- Chlamydia
- Gonorrhea
- Hepatitis B
- Herpes simplex virus (HSV)
- Human immunodeficiency viruses (HIV)
- Human papillomavirus (HPV)
- Syphilis
- Trichomoniasis

Of these eight STIs, four are curable. These four infections accounted for an estimated 376 million cases—or one in four new infections—in 2016:

- Chlamydia—127 million
- Gonorrhea—87 million
- Syphilis—6.3 million
- Trichomoniasis—156 million

The other four STIs—hepatitis B, HIV, HPV, and HSV—are caused by viruses and are incurable, although symptoms can be reduced or managed with treatment. Hepatitis B and HPV infections are preventable through vaccination.

Many STIs can be transmitted from mother to child, either during pregnancy or in childbirth. These STIs include the following:

- Chlamydia
- Gonorrhea
- Hepatitis B
- Herpes
- HIV
- HPV
- Syphilis

STI counseling and behavioral interventions, including comprehensive sex education, condom promotion, and risk-reduction counseling, are the primary ways STIs can be prevented. A lack of training for health workers, a lack of public awareness about the risks and symptoms of STIs, and continued stigma related to sex and STIs are the biggest obstacles to the effectiveness of STI interventions.

Question: What is the difference between HIV and AIDS?

Answer: First identified in 1981, HIV (human immunodeficiency virus) is a virus that attacks the cells that help the body fight infection, thus making the body more vulnerable to other infections and diseases. HIV is spread by contact with the bodily fluids of a person with the virus. Currently, there is no cure for HIV, so once a person has the virus, it stays in the body for the rest of that individual's life.

AIDS (acquired immunodeficiency syndrome) is the late stage of HIV infection, which occurs when the body's immune system has been badly compromised by the virus.

HIV medicine, known as ART (antiretroviral therapy), can help stop the progression of the HIV virus and prevent the development of AIDS.

Question: When and where do scientists think HIV likely originated?

Answer: HIV developed as a mutated version of a chimpanzee virus called simian immunodeficiency virus (SIV). Forensic experts analyzed mutations in the archived samples of HIV's genetic code to trace the evolutionary history of the virus. They concluded that HIV originated in the 1920s in the city of Kinshasa (Leopoldville until 1966), in what is now the Democratic Republic of the Congo.

It is believed that the chimpanzee version of the virus—SIV—made the jump from chimpanzees to humans because chimpanzees were hunted for meat. Handling and consuming infected blood transmitted the chimpanzee virus to humans, where SIV mutated into HIV.

The earliest known case of an HIV-1 infection in humans was found in a 1959 blood sample that had been collected from a man in Kinshasa—but how he became infected with HIV remains unknown.

The hunting of chimpanzees for meat contributed to the simian version of the virus mutating into the human virus HIV, but rapid population growth, unclean practices in health clinics, and a large sex trade led to the virus slowly spreading throughout the region—and, eventually, into other parts of the world.

Question: Where were the first cases of HIV/AIDS identified in the United States?

Answer: Scientists believe HIV spread from Africa to Haiti and the Caribbean in the 1960s when Haitian professionals returned home from the colonial Democratic Republic of the Congo. HIV then spread to New York City from the Caribbean around 1970, and from there it spread to San Francisco around a decade later. International travel from the United States contributed to the spread of the virus to other parts of the world.

In 1980, San Francisco resident Ken Horne became the first recognized case of HIV/AIDS in the United States. However, in 1987 molecular biologists at Tulane University tested samples of the remains of Robert Rayford, a Black teenager from St. Louis, Missouri, and found evidence of HIV. The teenager, referenced as Robert R. due to his age, admitted himself to the hospital in early 1968 with an array of symptoms that puzzled doctors.

Following the death of the sixteen-year-old from pneumonia in May 1969, an autopsy revealed several abnormalities, including lesions related to Kaposi's sarcoma, a rare type of cancer that would later be designated as an AIDS-defining illness. Rayford had never traveled outside the Midwest or received a blood transfusion, leading doctors to speculate he may have been exposed to the virus as a child prostitute. Because he stated that he had been experiencing symptoms since late 1966, Rayford may be the earliest case of HIV/AIDS in the United States.

Question: **How did HIV and AIDS get their names, and when was HIV first identified as the virus that causes AIDS?**

Answer: Because HIV does not have noticeable symptoms, the virus continued to spread in Africa, and eventually into other parts of the world, while remaining unknown until the 1980s. In 1981, the CDC published a paper about five healthy homosexual men in Los Angeles who had become infected with *Pneumocystis carinii*, a strain of pneumonia that rarely affects people with uncompromised immune systems.

As the number of cases of this new immune system disorder grew, it was initially called gay-related immune deficiency, or GRID, because the people who seemed to be most affected were gay men. Eventually, the CDC identified the routes of disease transmission, including heterosexual contact, and in September 1982, began calling the disease acquired immunodeficiency syndrome, or AIDS.

In 1983, scientists discovered the virus that causes AIDS. The virus was variously referred to as HTLV-III/LAV (human T-cell lymphotropic virus-type III/lymphadenopathy-associated virus), and AIDS-associated retrovirus (ARV). After a year of deliberating over the name, the Retrovirus Study Group of the International Committee on Taxonomy of Viruses (ICTV) settled on human immunodeficiency virus, or HIV, in 1986.

Question: How has HIV/AIDS been portrayed in the media and pop culture?

Answer: Initially believed to affect only homosexual men, AIDS was first referred to as gay-related immune deficiency, or GRID. Although researchers soon realized that anyone could become infected with HIV/AIDS, the illness disproportionately affected the homosexual community and as a result was referred to as the "gay plague" or the "gay disease."

In 1985, actor Rock Hudson became the first high-profile person to die of AIDS—and his death was the first of many AIDS-related deaths in the entertainment and sports communities. Throughout the next three decades, the HIV/AIDS epidemic would affect popular culture in profound ways, helping to change the perception of the illness and the people it affected. These are some highlights:

- *1985*: NBC airs the TV movie *An Early Frost*, starring Aidan Quinn as a gay, HIV-positive Chicago lawyer, just one month after Rock Hudson's death. The drama earns fourteen Emmy nominations that year, winning four.

- **1987**: The AIDS Coalition to Unleash Power—ACT UP—forms, organizing public protests to raise awareness about the AIDS crisis.

- **1993**: Tom Hanks wins a Best Actor Academy Award for his performance in *Philadelphia*. Hanks plays Andrew Beckett, a gay corporate attorney who is fired when his coworkers learn he has AIDS.

- **1993**: *Angels in America*, Tony Kushner's play about the AIDS epidemic, wins the Pulitzer Prize for Drama.

- **1994**: The musical *RENT* reinterprets *La Bohème*, Puccini's opera about the nineteenth century tuberculosis epidemic, as a story about artists and performers living in New York City during the Reagan-era AIDS crisis.

- **1994**: Reality television series *The Real World: San Francisco* features Pedro Zamora, a gay Cuban immigrant with HIV. Zamora, who becomes one of the series' most popular characters, dies shortly after the show's season finale.

- **1996**: The novel *Push* by Sapphire tells the story of sixteen-year-old Claireece "Precious" Jones, who becomes pregnant and infected with HIV after she is raped by her father. The book is later adapted into the 2009 film *Precious*, which receives six Academy Award nominations, winning two.

- **2000**: The American television drama *Queer as Folk* is the first show to portray contemporary life in the gay and lesbian community and feature regular storylines centering on HIV/AIDS.

- **2003**: South Africa's *Takalani Sesame*, a project modeled after *Sesame Street*, introduces Kami, the first HIV-positive Muppet, offering facts about HIV and AIDS and showing that touching and playing with those who are HIV-positive is okay.
- **2004**: The HBO miniseries adaptation of *Angels in America* wins a record number of Emmy awards, taking home eleven awards, including Outstanding Miniseries.

Question: **Is there a cure for HIV? Will there ever be a cure?**

Answer: There is currently no cure for HIV. Once the infection has been acquired, it remains in the body forever. But antiretroviral therapy (ART) can control HIV and prevent complications from developing, allowing people to live long and healthy lives.

ART involves taking a combination of three or more medications from different drug classes, often in the form of one pill taken once daily for the rest of the individual's life. Although ART does not cure HIV, this combination approach to drug treatment lowers the amount of HIV in the blood.

Scientists continue to research a cure for HIV, focusing on two types of cures:

- *A functional cure would suppress the HIV virus in the body to an undetectable level.* Although HIV would still be present in the body, it would not cause illness. This is similar to antiretroviral therapy, but a functional cure would suppress the virus without the need for ongoing ART treatment. A few people have been considered functionally cured after receiving ART shortly after birth or after infection, but the virus reemerged in all the cases.

- *A sterilizing cure would eradicate the virus from the body.* So far, only two people are known to have been cured this way. In 2007–08, Timothy Brown, an American living in Berlin, Germany, received a bone marrow transplant to treat leukemia. The transplant came from someone with a natural genetic resistance to HIV, which cured Brown's HIV. Scientists don't yet understand why Brown was cured, but the results have given researchers information they can use as they work to cure HIV. Brown died in September 2020 following a recurrence of leukemia. Adam Castillejo, a patient in London, became the second person believed to have been cured as a result of a bone marrow transplant in 2016.

Question: Will there ever be an HIV vaccine?

Answer: A vaccine to protect against HIV does not yet exist, but trials are under way for different HIV vaccines— and several of them have demonstrated encouraging results. A successful HIV vaccine likely won't be available until 2030—nearly fifty years after AIDS was identified.

Because vaccines have historically proven to be the most effective way to prevent infectious disease, researchers believe an HIV vaccine could be the safest and most cost-effective way to prevent illness and death caused by HIV/AIDS. However, an HIV vaccine would likely offer only partial protection against the virus and would therefore need to be used in conjunction with other prevention and treatment options.

Question: **Is HIV/AIDS still a global health concern?**

Answer: Worldwide, the spread of HIV peaked in 1996, and the number of AIDS-related deaths peaked in 2004. However, HIV/AIDS remains a major health concern, especially across sub-Saharan Africa, and is still one of the world's most fatal infectious diseases.

Misinformation about how HIV/AIDS is transmitted and a lack of public awareness of the disease, along with the stigma surrounding homosexuality, contributed to the spread of HIV/AIDS. The first cases reported by the CDC in 1981 signaled the beginning of a global epidemic, with reported cases of AIDS increasing dramatically in the United States. Around the world, approximately 76 million people have become infected since the start of the epidemic.

Worldwide, there were around 38 million people with HIV/AIDS in 2019, with 1.7 million new infections. Since 2010, new HIV infections have dropped by 23 percent, and since the 2004 peak, AIDS-related deaths have been reduced by 60 percent.

In the United States, around 1.2 million people are living with HIV, and about 14 percent—or one in seven—of those people do not know they are infected. In 2018, there were 37,968 new HIV diagnoses and 17,032 new AIDS diagnoses.

Although progress has been made in reducing the global number of HIV/AIDS cases, it continues to be a significant public health issue.

CHAPTER 7

INFECTIOUS DISEASES AROUND THE WORLD

What We Know About the
Global Impact of Disease

Question: What are tropical diseases, and why do they occur in warmer parts of the world?

Answer: In comparison to more temperate areas of the world, tropical geographic regions have historically been more affected by infectious diseases because, owing to a combination of biological and environmental factors, bacteria, parasites, and viruses thrive in warm, humid climates.

Tropical infectious diseases include the following:

- Arboviruses (including West Nile virus and Zika virus)
- Cholera
- Dengue fever
- Ebola virus
- Lassa virus
- Malaria
- Tuberculosis
- Yellow fever

Question: What are diseases of poverty and neglected tropical diseases?

Answer: Diseases of poverty are those that affect the poorest populations at a disproportionately higher rate—and many of these illnesses are infectious diseases. Although all types of bacteria, fungi, parasites, and viruses that cause infectious diseases can be found worldwide, it is people in poverty who suffer the most.

The three primary diseases of poverty are HIV/AIDS, malaria, and tuberculosis. These diseases account for 18 percent of diseases in poor countries and 10 percent of global mortality.

Other diseases that fall under the umbrella of diseases of poverty include a number of neglected tropical diseases, or NTDs. Neglected tropical diseases are communicable parasitic and bacterial diseases that affect more than one billion people globally. The world's poorest populations are most affected by these diseases, which affect physical and cognitive development, as well as mother and child mortality. NTDs create a cycle of poverty and disease that is difficult for communities to escape.

As of 2017, the World Health Organization has categorized twenty neglected tropical diseases:

- Buruli ulcer
- Chagas disease (American trypanosomiasis)
- Cysticercosis
- Dengue
- Dracunculiasis (Guinea worm disease)
- Echinococcosis
- Endemic treponematoses (including yaws)
- Foodborne trematode infections
- HIV/AIDS
- Human African trypanosomiasis (sleeping sickness)
- Leishmaniasis
- Leprosy
- Lymphatic filariasis (elephantiasis)
- Malaria
- Onchocerciasis (river blindness)
- Rabies
- Schistosomiasis (bilharziasis)
- Soil-transmitted helminth (intestinal parasitic worms) infections
- Trachoma
- Tuberculosis

Six of these NTDs can be controlled or eliminated through mass drug administration or other interventions, including controlling insect vectors and improving hygiene and sanitation practices.

These are the six NTDs that can be controlled or eliminated:

- Dracunculiasis (Guinea worm disease)
- Lymphatic filariasis (elephantiasis)
- Onchocerciasis (river blindness)
- Schistosomiasis (bilharziasis)
- Soil-transmitted helminth (STH) infections (including infections from *Ascaris*, hookworm, and whipworm)
- Trachoma

Question: **How has the advent of air travel affected the spread of infectious diseases?**

Answer: Commercial aviation has been around for about a century, but it became increasingly popular following World War II. Now, more than two billion people travel by air each year, providing many opportunities to see the world, get jet lag—and contribute to the spread of infectious diseases.

Anyone who has ever traveled by airplane has likely had the occasion to consider the risk of contracting an illness from their fellow travelers. And anyone who has ever had "travel crud" knows just how easily sickness can spread.

An infectious disease can be transmitted on an aircraft in a variety of ways, including the following:

- Close contact with large droplets
- Airborne spread through small-particle aerosols
- Contaminated food
- The transport of infected animals or insects

The actual risk of infectious disease transmission on a commercial aircraft is generally unknown due to insufficient historical data and a number of uncontrolled variables. However, researchers have documented in-flight transmission of infectious diseases on commercial aircraft, including the following:

- Cholera
- Influenza
- Measles
- Meningococcal infections
- Norovirus
- Severe acute respiratory syndrome (SARS)
- Tuberculosis

An investigation of in-flight transmission of tuberculosis showed that the greatest risk of transmission occurs when sitting within two rows of a contagious passenger on a flight longer than eight hours.

Question: **What is Ebola virus, and where does it get its name?**

Answer: Ebola virus disease (EVD) is one of the world's deadliest viral diseases. It was discovered in 1976 after two consecutive outbreaks of fatal hemorrhagic fever occurred in different parts of central Africa. Also known as Ebola hemorrhagic fever, the first recorded outbreak occurred in a village in the Democratic Republic of the Congo (formerly Zaire) near the Ebola River, giving the virus its name. The second outbreak occurred at the same time, but around five hundred miles away in what is now South Sudan.

Initially, it was believed that the two outbreaks were actually a single event linked by an infected person who had traveled between the two locations. Scientists eventually discovered that the outbreaks were caused by two genetically distinct viruses, which they named *Zaire ebolavirus* (ZEBOV) and *Sudan ebolavirus* (SUDV).

Other species in the genus *Ebolavirus* (EBOV) include *Bundibugyo ebolavirus*, *Taï Forest ebolavirus*, *Reston ebolavirus*, and *Bombali ebolavirus*. Of the six identified species of *Ebolavirus*, only four—*Zaire*, *Sudan*, *Taï Forest*, and *Bundibugyo*—are known to cause diseases in people. Of the other two species, *Reston ebolavirus* can cause disease in pigs and nonhuman primates but not people, and it's not yet known whether *Bombali ebolavirus*, which was identified in bats in 2018, can cause disease in people or animals.

Of the *Ebolavirus* species, all but *Reston ebolavirus* have been detected exclusively in Africa. *Reston ebolavirus* was first isolated in 1989–90 in Reston, Virginia, from macaques (monkeys) that had been imported from the Philippines. In 2008, pigs imported from the Philippines also tested positive for *Reston ebolavirus*.

Ebola virus is considered to be an emerging zoonotic disease that most commonly affects humans and nonhuman primates (such as apes, chimpanzees, and monkeys), with fruit bats being natural hosts. The virus initially spreads through direct contact with the blood, bodily fluids, and tissues of infected animals, getting in through mucous membranes in the nose, mouth, or eyes, or through broken skin. The disease can then spread from person to person through direct contact with the bodily fluids of a person who is sick or has died from the virus. The Ebola virus can linger in certain bodily fluids, such as semen, making sexual transmission possible even after a person has recovered from EVD.

Symptoms of Ebola virus appear two to twenty-one days after infection and can include the following:

- Headache
- High fever
- Joint and muscle aches
- Lack of appetite
- Sore throat
- Stomach pain
- Weakness

Data suggest that Ebola virus existed before the 1976 outbreaks. Population growth, human encroachment on forests, and human interaction with wildlife are all implicated in the spread of this virus.

Following the discovery of Ebola virus disease in 1976, occasional outbreaks of the virus occurred, most often in remote rainforests of central and East Africa. But in 2013, West Africa experienced an outbreak that began in a rural area of southeastern Guinea and quickly spread across the borders of Sierra Leone and Liberia and into densely populated urban areas, sparking an epidemic that lasted from 2014 until 2016.

Another outbreak of EVD began in the Democratic Republic of the Congo in 2018. Both the 2014–16 and 2018–19 Ebola virus outbreaks were of the *Zaire ebolavirus* species. Currently, several Ebola vaccines are being tested in clinical trials around the world, but no licensed vaccine to prevent Ebola virus disease exists yet.

Question: Have there been any cases of Ebola virus disease in the United States?

Answer: In 2014, the year an outbreak of Ebola virus disease (EVD) began surging throughout parts of West Africa, there were eleven documented cases of Ebola virus in the United States. Nine of those cases were individuals who had contracted the disease outside the United States before traveling into the country, either as medical evacuees or as commercial airline passengers. Of those nine people, two of them died as a result of the illness: Thomas Eric Duncan, who traveled from Liberia to visit family in Texas, and Martin Salia, MD, who was a medical evacuee from Sierra Leone. Duncan was the first confirmed case of Ebola in the United States.

The two people who became infected with Ebola virus in the United States were both nurses treating Duncan at Texas Health Presbyterian Hospital in Dallas. Both made a full recovery from the illness.

Question: Why is it called yellow fever?

Answer: Yellow fever takes its name from one of the symptoms of the toxic phase of the illness—jaundice, or the yellowing of the skin. But not all people reach this level of infection.

Found in tropical and subtropical areas of Africa and South America, yellow fever is a mosquito-borne infection also referred to as yellow jack, black vomit, or American plague. Yellow fever has an acute phase and sometimes a toxic phase. Following an incubation period that lasts three to six days, a person enters the acute stage, which has a range of symptoms, including fever, headache, body aches, light sensitivity, loss of appetite, dizziness, and nausea.

In mild cases of yellow fever, people recover from the acute phase after several days. However, some people experience a toxic phase of the illness, which can be fatal. Symptoms of the toxic phase include jaundice as well as decreased urination; bleeding from the nose, eyes, and mouth; liver and kidney failure; slowed heart rate; abdominal pain and vomiting; and brain dysfunction, including delirium, seizures, and coma.

Because there is no specific treatment for yellow fever, physicians recommend that travelers receive a yellow fever vaccine before traveling to an area where there is a risk of exposure to the disease.

Question: **What does gin and tonic have to do with preventing malaria?**

Answer: In the early-nineteenth century, British officials stationed in tropical posts such as India were directed to dissolve quinine powder in carbonated tonic water to protect themselves against malaria.

Discovered in the eighteenth century by Scottish physician George Cleghorn to be an effective treatment for malaria, quinine is what gives tonic water its distinctive bitter taste. Drinking it in soda water—sometimes with sugar added—made it go down easier. Eventually, the British added gin to their medicinal quinine tonic water, creating the classic G&T cocktail.

Malaria is caused by the Plasmodium parasite, which gets into the red blood cells and causes sickness. Quinine doesn't actually prevent malaria—it kills the parasite or prevents it from growing.

Tonic water was also known as Indian tonic water and was first commercially produced in 1858. Today, tonic water contains far less quinine than the recommended therapeutic dose, so no, drinking gin and tonics will not protect someone from catching malaria.

Medicinal quinine is now prescribed in pill form.

Question: **Which insects transmit diseases, and what diseases do they transmit?**

Answer: Several insects act as vectors for transmitting infectious pathogens to humans and animals. The pathogens transmitted by these insects include bacteria, parasites, and viruses. Many of these vector-borne diseases are found in tropical and subtropical climates and disproportionately affect poor populations.

These are the insects that serve as agents for disease transmission, and some of the diseases they can transmit:

- *Aquatic snails*: Schistosomiasis (bilharziasis)
- *Blackflies*: Onchocerciasis (river blindness)
- *Fleas*: Plague (transmitted from rats to humans), tungiasis
- *Lice*: Typhus, louse-borne relapsing fever

- *Mosquitoes, Aedes species*: Chikungunya, dengue, lymphatic filariasis, Rift Valley fever, yellow fever, Zika
- *Mosquitoes, Anopheles species*: lymphatic filariasis, malaria
- *Mosquitoes, Culex species*: Japanese encephalitis, lymphatic filariasis, West Nile fever
- *Sandflies*: Leishmaniasis, sandfly fever (phlebotomus fever)
- *Ticks*: Crimean-Congo hemorrhagic fever, Lyme disease, relapsing fever (borreliosis), rickettsial diseases (spotted fever and Q fever), tick-borne encephalitis, tularemia
- *Triatomine bugs*: Chagas disease (American trypanosomiasis)
- *Tsetse flies*: Sleeping sickness (African trypanosomiasis)

Question: How did King Tut die?

Answer: A two-year DNA study conducted of ancient Egyptian royal mummies and published in 2010 gave researchers a better understanding of what probably killed King Tutankhamun. The frail nineteen-year-old boy pharaoh, who died around 1324 BCE, likely succumbed to a combination of disorders, including a degenerative bone condition, leg fracture, and severe malarial infection. There are no surviving records about the circumstances of Tut's death, so prior to the DNA study, scientists had only been able to guess about the cause of his early death. Over the years since the discovery of his mummy, there had been speculation that he might have been murdered by a blow to the head or even poison.

Instead, researchers found the DNA from several strains of the mosquito-borne parasite that causes malaria in King Tut's body. The presence of multiple strains indicated that the young pharaoh had been repeatedly infected with malaria tropica, the most severe strain of malaria. This discovery, found in four of the precisely dated mummies, including Tut's, is believed to mark the oldest genetic proof of the disease.

Examinations of King Tut's mummy have revealed a leg fracture as well as deformations in his left foot caused by necrosis of bone tissue. With his immune system weakened by repeated bouts of malaria, King Tut would have struggled to heal from his physical injuries.

CHAPTER 8

LIVING HISTORY

The Novel Coronavirus, the COVID-19 Pandemic, and the Future of Disease

Question: When will the COVID-19 pandemic end?

Answer: It's too early to know when COVID-19 will end. Historically, pandemics have both a medical and a social end, with the medical end coming after the rates of disease and mortality fall below the baseline of the disease and stay there, due to vaccination and also due to herd immunity being achieved.

Usually, the social end of a pandemic, when people feel it is safe to resume normal life, occurs after the medical end. But there are signs that the COVID-19 pandemic may have a social end before it reaches a medical conclusion, and that decisions about the "end" of the pandemic may be driven more by economic and political concerns rather than medical and public health data.

This is a concern because if a social end precedes a medical end, this suggests that people no longer fear the disease and its potential consequences—or it may signal that the population has learned to live with the disease and its consequences. Neither situation is ideal and can cause the disease to linger in the population, contributing to an increased number of illnesses and deaths.

Question: How did COVID-19 create a coin shortage?

Answer: The United States experienced an unusual consequence as a result of the COVID-19 pandemic—a national coin shortage.

Public spaces, where vending machines and laundromats are found, serve as large deposit centers for coins. These coins are then deposited in banks or traded in for paper bills, allowing the banks to recirculate the coins back to the public. Business and bank closures, as well as a reduction in traffic in the public spaces where coins typically accumulate, all contributed to a coin shortage due to a slowed pace of circulation, reducing available coin inventories.

In July 2020, the Federal Reserve created a US Coin Task Force to mitigate the situation by identifying, implementing, and promoting actions that addressed the coin shortage.

Question: **Did scientists predict the COVID-19 pandemic? Why weren't we ready?**

Answer: Experts who study zoonotic coronaviruses have been concerned for years about the potential for a human coronavirus pandemic. An October 2007 research paper published in *Clinical Microbiology Reviews* posits the following:

> *The presence of a large reservoir of SARS-CoV-like viruses in horseshoe bats, together with the culture of eating exotic mammals in southern China, is a time bomb. The possibility of the reemergence of SARS and other novel viruses from animals or laboratories and therefore the need for preparedness should not be ignored.*

Despite the early warnings that a coronavirus pandemic might be on the near horizon, skepticism about the potential risks and a lack of funding impeded the development of treatments and vaccines for SARS, which, due to the similarities between the coronaviruses, could have been relevant to the preparation of treatments for COVID-19.

Question: What is meant by the term *novel coronavirus*?

Answer: A novel coronavirus is a new coronavirus. There are many types of human coronaviruses (HCoVs). SARS-CoV-2, which causes COVID-19 disease, is a new (or novel) coronavirus that started in an animal population and had not been previously identified in humans.

The name *coronavirus* refers to what the virus looks like under an electron microscope. All coronaviruses have a similar structure and are named for the "corona," or crown-like spikes, on their surface. There are four main coronavirus groups: alpha, beta, gamma, and delta.

Question: Why is it called COVID-19? Why do the virus and the disease have different names?

Answer: Viruses often have names that are different from the diseases they cause. COVID-19 is the official name for the disease caused by the 2019 novel coronavirus first reported in Wuhan, China, on December 31, 2019. *CO* stands for "corona," *VI* for "virus," and *D* for "disease," while *19* refers to the year the disease was first identified.

Diseases are named by the World Health Organization in the International Classification of Diseases. Naming diseases is important for facilitating discussions about disease prevention, spread, and treatment.

The novel coronavirus that causes COVID-19 was first known as 2019-nCoV before being renamed SARS-CoV-2, or severe acute respiratory syndrome coronavirus 2. SARS-CoV-2 shares a genetic link with the coronavirus that caused the 2003 SARS outbreak, but despite their genetic relationship, the SARS-CoV-2 virus is different from its SARS predecessor.

Question: How did COVID-19 start?

Answer: The outbreak of a novel coronavirus disease was first identified on December 31, 2019, in Wuhan, China. Epidemiologists did field investigations by conducting surveys and collecting nose and throat specimens from people in the area where the coronavirus was initially detected. Through these investigations, the scientists were able to determine who was infected, when they became sick, and where they had been before falling ill. With this information, doctors speculated that the novel coronavirus had a zoonotic source and may have come from an animal sold at a market.

As of September 2020, researchers were still not certain which animal might have transmitted SARS-CoV-2 to humans. Several studies suggest that SARS-CoV-2 is the result of a cross-species evolution between two animal species, originating in horseshoe bats and jumping to humans by way of an intermediary, the pangolin, a nocturnal anteater. This animal is illegally poached and sold for both medicinal products and meat, and is the most trafficked mammal in the world.

Question: What's the difference between the virus that causes COVID-19 and previously identified coronaviruses?

Answer: SARS-CoV-2, the virus that causes COVID-19, is part of the coronavirus family, a group of viruses that cause a variety of respiratory illnesses, such as the common cold, Middle East respiratory syndrome (MERS), and severe acute respiratory syndrome (SARS).

The main difference between previously identified coronaviruses and SARS-CoV-2 is that the novel coronavirus hasn't been seen in humans before. This means that humans haven't yet developed a natural immunity to this particular strain of coronavirus, nor do we have an effective vaccine yet.

SARS-CoV-2 also appears to be more contagious than other human coronaviruses (HCoVs), likely due to the fact that it is a new virus and the human immune system isn't prepared to fight it. It's too early to tell what COVID-19's public health impact will be in the long term. Some researchers believe COVID-19, like the seasonal flu, might stay with us.

Question: **What are the similarities and differences between the novel coronavirus and influenza viruses?**

Answer: The novel coronavirus SARS-CoV-2 and influenza viruses share some similarities, which can make it hard to tell the difference between them based only on symptoms. Testing may be necessary to confirm a diagnosis.

Both COVID-19 and influenza cause respiratory disease, which presents as a wide range of illness, from asymptomatic or mild disease to severe disease and even death. Both viruses are transmitted by close person-to-person contact, and are spread mainly by droplets formed when an infected person sneezes, coughs, or even talks. These droplets then land on the mouths or noses of people nearby (generally within six feet) and can be inhaled into the lungs.

Both COVID-19 and influenza viruses can also be transmitted by physical person-to-person contact, such as shaking hands or touching a surface that has the virus on it and transferring it to the mouth, nose, or even eyes.

For both COVID-19 and influenza, frequent handwashing, covering one's cough, disposing of tissues immediately after use, staying home when sick, and limiting contact with people who are, or may be, infected are all effective actions in helping to reduce and prevent the spread of infection.

These are common symptoms caused by both COVID-19 and influenza viruses:

- Chills
- Cough
- Fatigue
- Fever (or feeling feverish)
- Headache
- Muscle pain or body aches
- Runny or stuffy nose
- Shortness of breath or difficulty breathing
- Sore throat
- Vomiting and diarrhea (more common in children than adults)

One notable difference in symptoms is that COVID-19 may cause a change in or loss of sense of taste or smell.

Another reason testing to confirm a diagnosis of COVID-19 or influenza is important is that symptoms of COVID-19 can take longer to develop than symptoms of influenza. Flu symptoms typically develop within one to four days after infection, while COVID-19 symptoms typically develop anywhere from two to fourteen days after infection, although typically it's around five days before symptoms appear. A person with COVID-19 can also be contagious for a longer period of time than someone with the flu.

Both COVID-19 and influenza can cause severe illness and complications for people in high-risk categories, including people with certain comorbidities, older adults, and pregnant people. The risk of severe illness and complications for healthy children with no underlying medical conditions appears to be higher for influenza than COVID-19.

With both COVID-19 and influenza, complications can include the following:

- Acute respiratory distress syndrome
- Heart attack, stroke, or other cardiac injury
- Inflammation of the heart, brain, or muscle tissues
- Multiple-organ failure (respiratory failure, kidney failure, and shock)
- Pneumonia
- Respiratory failure
- Secondary bacterial infections
- Sepsis
- Worsening of chronic medical conditions (diabetes or those medical conditions that involve the lungs, heart, or nervous system)

COVID-19 can cause additional complications, including blood clots in the arteries and veins of the lungs, brain, heart, or legs. Children infected with COVID-19 are also at higher risk of a rare but severe complication that causes multisystem inflammatory syndrome in children.

The biggest difference between COVID-19 and influenza is that COVID-19 is a novel virus that researchers and scientists are still learning about while influenza viruses are familiar and well studied. Several licensed influenza vaccines are produced every year to protect against the influenza viruses that scientists anticipate will circulate that year. Although researchers and vaccine developers are currently working at a rapid pace to create a vaccine that will prevent COVID-19, such a vaccine is not yet available.

Question: **What is the test for COVID-19?**

Answer: There are currently two tests available for diagnosing a COVID-19 infection:

- A viral test, which identifies a current COVID-19 infection
- An antibody test, which can identify that a previous infection has occurred

An antibody test may not be able to identify a current infection because it can take one to three weeks after an infection to develop the antibodies. Having antibodies to the virus that causes COVID-19 might help provide protection from becoming reinfected by the virus, although researchers don't yet know how much protection the antibodies might provide or how long that protection will last.

Question: What are comorbidities?

Answer: Comorbidities may also be called coexisting or co-occurring conditions or referred to as multimorbidity or multiple chronic conditions.

The term *comorbidity* was first used in the 1970s by physician and epidemiologist A. R. Feinstein. A comorbidity occurs when more than one disease or condition is present in the same person at the same time. Conditions described as comorbidities are often chronic or long-term conditions that can affect how a person experiences a new disease or infection. In describing comorbidity, Feinstein used the example of people with rheumatic fever, who often have multiple other diseases.

Although it isn't unusual for people to experience two chronic illnesses at once, comorbidities can worsen the outcome and lead to additional complications of an infectious disease. Comorbidities can also complicate the treatment plan for an infectious disease.

Question: What is contact tracing?

Answer: In public health, contact tracing is the process of identifying people who may have come into contact with a person who has an infectious disease. Tracing the contacts of infected people allows those contacts to be tested, isolated, and treated for the infection they have been exposed to.

Contact tracing is used for infectious diseases, including vaccine-preventable infections, such as measles; sexually transmitted infections, including HIV; tuberculosis; Ebola virus disease; blood-borne infections; serious bacterial infections; and novel infections, including H1N1, SARS-CoV, and SARS-CoV-2, the novel virus that causes COVID-19.

These are the goals of contact tracing:

- To interrupt the ongoing transmission of infection and reduce its spread
- To alert contacts of the possibility of infection and provide them with preventive or prophylactic services
- To provide diagnosis, treatment, and counseling to those people who are already infected
- To prevent reinfection of the original infected patient if the infection is treatable
- To learn about how a disease affects a particular population

Question: **How can technology be used to manage contact tracing?**

Answer: Smartphones can aid in contact tracing by providing proximity information using GPS, Bluetooth, or Wi-Fi signals.

Contact tracing software for COVID-19 has been developed and introduced in Canada and several European countries. Digital tracking technology, although an effective means of contact tracing, can also have privacy issues associated with it. For this reason, technology is not yet a reliable method of contact tracing.

In August 2020, Virginia became the first state to use new pandemic technology created by a collaboration between Apple and Google. Covidwise is a smartphone app that can automatically notify people if they might have been exposed to COVID-19.

Available for both Apple and Android smartphones, Covidwise is a free app that uses Bluetooth wireless technology to detect when two phones come into close proximity. People who test positive for COVID-19 can update their testing status via their phone and anonymously notify other smartphone users they've come into contact with about potential exposure. Those who are warned about possible exposure to COVID-19 can then pursue advice and testing through their doctor or state health department.

The Covidwise app defines close contact as being within six feet of someone for at least fifteen minutes. People separated by a wall (such as in a dormitory or office building) might still receive a notification of potential exposure, depending on the Bluetooth signal strength.

Question: **Can we use the pandemic flu of 1918 as a model for what to expect from COVID-19?**

Answer: During a public health crisis, such as the COVID-19 pandemic, looking to the past can give researchers and scientists insights into how to proceed— but historical data provided by an influenza pandemic cannot be used to determine how to manage a novel coronavirus.

Because COVID-19 shares some basic similarities with influenza viruses, researchers have been guided by the 1918 influenza pandemic with regard to promoting policies and interventions designed to mitigate the spread of the virus. However, it's not possible to use the 1918 flu pandemic to make comparisons or predictions about the COVID-19 pandemic because the two viruses that caused the pandemics are biologically different. Researchers believe that because of mutations in SARS-CoV-2, the virus that causes COVID-19, the predictable "waves" of disease that were experienced with the H1N1 virus of 1918 are unlikely to occur with COVID-19.

Historically, the 1918 pandemic ebbed, despite the lack of an influenza vaccine, following a third wave in the spring of 1919. But the wave pattern and eventual fading of the H1N1 virus that caused the 1918 pandemic cannot be used to predict the outcome of COVID-19.

Question: **How long will it take for a COVID-19 vaccine to become available?**

Answer: Scientists don't know how long it will take to develop a vaccine to protect against the novel coronavirus, SARS-CoV-2, which causes COVID-19.

Vaccine research and development is a long, thorough multistep process. It can take ten to fifteen years to move through the phases of development to license a safe, effective vaccine—and it can cost as much as 500 million dollars to get there.

Even with community measures to reduce the spread of the virus, such as social distancing, contact tracing, and mask wearing, the novel coronavirus (SARS-CoV-2) that causes COVID-19 is likely to be with us for a long time—making the need for a vaccine even more crucial. But there has never been a coronavirus vaccine for humans before, which contributes to the uncertainty of how quickly a vaccine may be available. The fastest vaccine ever developed was for mumps, and that took four years.

It helps that scientists didn't have to start from scratch with regard to COVID-19 vaccine research. Middle East respiratory syndrome (MERS) and severe acute respiratory syndrome (SARS) are also caused by coronaviruses, with SARS and SARS-CoV-2 being around 8 percent identical, which is why scientists were able to quickly develop a test for COVID-19 and begin working on a possible vaccine.

By the summer of 2020, there were almost one hundred vaccines in various stages of development and dozens of vaccines were starting clinical trials. But the reality is that less than 10 percent of drugs that reach the clinical trial stage are approved by the Food and Drug Administration.

Through a global effort of scientists and researchers moving as quickly as possible through the vaccine development process, it's possible that an effective COVID-19 vaccine could be available to the public in twelve to eighteen months—sometime in 2021. But experts caution that this may be an overly ambitious timeline. Stay tuned.

Question: What is Operation Warp Speed?

Answer: Introduced in April 2020, Operation Warp Speed (OWS) is a public-private partnership among several agencies of the US Department of Health and Human Services (HHS), including the Centers for Disease Control and Prevention (CDC), the Food and Drug Administration (FDA), the National Institutes of Health (NIH), the Biomedical Advanced Research and Development

Authority (BARDA), and the Department of Defense (DoD), as well as other federal agencies and private firms.

The collaborative purpose of OWS is to facilitate and accelerate the development, production, and distribution of COVID-19 vaccines, therapies, and diagnostics, with a goal of delivering three hundred million doses of a safe, effective COVID-19 vaccine by January 2021.

Question: **Why was COVID-19 called the Wuhan virus and the Chinese virus before it was called COVID-19?**

Answer: Naming a novel virus is a complicated process that isn't without controversy. When news of the novel coronavirus first broke, there was a need to give it a name—fast—in order to report on it.

The novel coronavirus, initially known as 2019-nCoV, was eventually renamed SARS-Cov-2, but the jumble of letters and numbers can be confusing for the general public. Articles began referring to the virus in relation to where it was first identified—the Wuhan virus, the China virus, the Chinese virus, the Wu Flu.

Such place names not only lead to confusion but contribute to prejudice and discrimination against specific groups of people and regions of the world.

The World Health Organization (WHO) has guidelines for best naming practices for new infectious diseases. The name should not offend any cultural, ethnic, national, professional, regional, or social group, and its impact on trade, travel, tourism, and animal welfare should be as minimal as possible.

CHAPTER 9

INFECTIOUS DISEASES AND PANDEMICS IN POP CULTURE

Why We're Entertained by Illness—And What We Can Learn from the Movies

Question: Who is Anthony Fauci, MD?

Answer: Anthony Fauci, MD, is an American physician and immunologist who has served as the director of the National Institute of Allergy and Infectious Disease (NIAID) since 1984. The NIAID is one of the twenty-seven institutions and centers of the National Institutes of Health (NIH), which operates as an agency of the United States Department of Health and Human Services (HHS).

As a physician with the NIH, Fauci has advised six US presidents on domestic and global health issues for more than fifty years. A leading researcher during the AIDS epidemic in the 1980s, Fauci was a principal architect of the President's Emergency Plan for AIDS Relief, a program that has helped save millions of lives worldwide.

Since January 2020, Fauci has served as a lead member of the White House Coronavirus Task Force, which addresses the COVID-19 pandemic in the United States. His frequent appearances as a public health spokesperson during the COVID-19 pandemic have made him one of the most recognizable people in the nation and have led to him becoming somewhat of a pop culture icon.

During an appearance on CNN's *New Day*, when asked which actor should play him on TV, Fauci jokingly replied, "Oh, Brad Pitt, of course." The offhand comment led to the Academy Award–winning actor depicting Fauci on a *Saturday Night Live* skit—and earned Pitt an Emmy nomination for the performance.

Fauci was asked to throw out the first pitch of the Washington Nationals' season opening game against the New York Yankees. When baseball card company Topps issued a limited-edition trading card commemorating the event, the twenty-four-hour sale set an all-time record, with 51,512 cards being sold.

Question: **Is there really a horror movie about the COVID-19 pandemic?**

Answer: Not exactly. *Host*, released in August 2020 by streaming service Shudder, is a British found footage (that is, footage presented as though it were discovered, not created, by the filmmaker) horror movie that centers on the type of video conferencing so many people have become familiar with during the pandemic stay-at-home orders.

Host is the brainchild of director and cowriter Rob Savage. What started as a short prank video about a zombie in the attic became a viral video on Twitter and then inspired a movie about a remote séance that goes horribly wrong when a group of friends connect with an evil spirit.

The entire film was made in twelve weeks, with everyone from actors to stunt performers to special effects experts working from home. The end result is a one-of-a-kind horror movie that taps into the boredom, fear, and isolation of being on lockdown during a pandemic.

Question: Does the song "A Spoonful of Sugar" in *Mary Poppins* reference a particular disease?

Answer: The 1964 Walt Disney film *Mary Poppins* stars Julie Andrews as a magical British nanny who sings to her young charges:

> *A spoonful of sugar helps the medicine go down,*
>> *The medicine go down,*
>> *The medicine go down.*
> *Just a spoonful of sugar helps the medicine go down,*
>> *In a most delightful way!*

The song was penned by the Sherman Brothers, Robert Sherman and Richard Sherman, an American songwriting duo who wrote more musical film scores than any other songwriting team in history.

Robert Sherman got the idea for the song's lyrics from his own children. He arrived home one day to learn that the kids had received their polio vaccine. Believing that the vaccine had been administered as a shot, he asked whether it had hurt, but one of his children explained that the medicine had been given as a drop of liquid on a sugar cube. With that explanation, a song was born.

Although Jonas Salk's injectable polio vaccine was first introduced in 1955, his rival, Albert Sabin, developed an oral polio vaccine that became available in the United States in 1961. Salk's vaccine was based on an inactivated (dead) form of the virus while Sabin's vaccine used a weakened form of the virus, which triggered the body's immune system to produce antibodies against the active virus.

The Sabin oral vaccine is still used in many areas of the world, especially in economically underdeveloped countries. Due to its greater safety, the Salk injectable vaccine is the one currently approved for use in the United States. Despite their professional rivalry, Salk and Sabin together are responsible for the near-eradication of polio in the world. But only one of them inspired a song!

Question: **Why were blood tests once required before a marriage license could be issued?**

Answer: During the 1930s, the increasing rates of syphilis in the United States were the catalyst behind US Surgeon General Thomas Parran Jr.'s nationwide campaign to educate people about venereal disease, which we now call sexually transmitted infection.

In the name of hygiene and public health, states began passing laws that required couples applying for a marriage license to submit to a blood test, the stated purpose of which was to avoid the spread of venereal disease, such as syphilis, to a new spouse or cause birth defects in future children.

By 1944, thirty states had enacted mandatory premarital blood test laws. When syphilis rates dropped nationwide (but not necessarily because of the premarital blood tests), some states shifted the purpose of premarital blood tests to check for other diseases, including tuberculosis, rubella, and more recently, HIV.

As it turned out, mandatory premarital blood tests did little to halt the spread of disease and proved to be a deterrent to getting married in those states that required a blood test. Many marriage-minded couples opted instead to go to a state that didn't require the blood test—or they simply didn't get married at all. In time, states began to abolish their premarital blood test laws. Montana was the last state to require a premarital blood test (for rubella). The law was repealed in 2019.

Question: Is flesh-eating bacteria a real thing?

Answer: Flesh-eating bacteria, or flesh-eating disease, is a very real, but thankfully rare, illness that most people have heard of—thanks to television and film dramatizations—called necrotizing fasciitis.

Fictional accounts of necrotizing fasciitis have appeared in TV medical dramas such as *Grey's Anatomy* and *House* and, most recently, three Chicago-based television dramas. In October 2019, *Chicago Fire*, *Chicago Med*, and *Chicago P.D.* highlighted necrotizing fasciitis during a three-hour crossover event titled "Infection."

Caused by a bacterial skin infection, the illness is treated with antibiotics and surgery. But even with treatment, one out of three people with the infection will die from it.

Researchers believe that group A *Streptococcus* (group A strep) is the most common cause of necrotizing fasciitis, although other bacteria can cause it as well. The bacteria most often enters the body through a break in the skin, such as by a cut, burn, insect bite, or surgical wound. Once in the body, the infection can spread rapidly, making early diagnosis and treatment crucial.

Early symptoms of necrotizing fasciitis can include the following:

- Fever
- Red, swollen, or warm area of the skin that spreads quickly
- Severe pain, even beyond the area of the body that is red, swollen, or warm

Later symptoms can include these:

- Blisters, black spots, or ulcers on the skin
- Changes in skin color
- Diarrhea or nausea
- Dizziness
- Fatigue
- Pus or oozing at the site of infection

Good wound care is the best way to prevent bacterial skin infection. A person with an open wound or skin infection should avoid hot tubs, swimming pools, and natural bodies of water, such as lakes, oceans, and rivers. Most cases of necrotizing fasciitis occur at random and rarely spread through person-to-person contact. Most people who get it have a weakened immune system due to other health issues, such as cancer, diabetes, kidney disease, or liver disease.

The CDC tracks necrotizing fasciitis cases that are caused by group A strep. Since 2010, there have been approximately 700 to 1,200 cases each year, although the CDC believes this is an underestimate.

Question: Why does the World Health Organization (WHO) have global public health days?

Answer: The purpose of the WHO's global public health campaigns is to raise awareness about health issues that affect the world. Although many health issues are recognized throughout the year, the WHO member states have mandated nine days and two weeks of every year to focus attention on specific health issues.

Of the nine days that the WHO uses to raise awareness about global public health issues, five of them focus on infectious diseases:

- March 24—World Tuberculosis Day
- April 14—World Chagas Disease Day
- April 25—World Malaria Day
- July 28—World Hepatitis Day
- December 1—World AIDS Day

Question: What trends has the COVID-19 pandemic inspired? Why?

Answer: For most of us, the COVID-19 pandemic has been our only experience with things such as stay-at-home orders and mask mandates. It seems natural that people would turn to activities that give them a sense of control over their circumstances and evoke a comforting sense of nostalgia.

Among the trends ushered in by the COVID-19 pandemic have been an increase in homely activities, such as bread baking. Not only did sales spike for shelf-stable foods, snacks, produce, and meat, but sales of flour and yeast also hit an unprecedented high in the weeks after the first stay-at-home orders were issued.

Another trend that saw a resurgence due to the COVID-19 pandemic was vegetable gardening, with people spurred by empty grocery shelves and fears that industrial agriculture might fail. The increased interest in edible gardens hearkens back to the victory gardens of World War I.

Time spent outdoors, whether gardening or exercising, has also increased with the pandemic. In June 2020, 49 percent of American adults reported spending more time outside than they had before the pandemic.

Question: **What do Christmas Seals have to do with tuberculosis?**

Answer: The American Lung Association's Christmas Seals program got its start as a fundraising campaign for a tuberculosis sanatorium.

In the early-twentieth century, when tuberculosis was the leading cause of death in the United States, doctors began having some success in treating tuberculosis patients at specialized hospitals known as sanatoriums.

In 1907, a Delaware sanatorium was experiencing financial troubles and needed to raise funds to continue to care for patients. Enterprising hospital volunteer Emily Bissell started a public campaign to raise funds by designing and printing holiday seals—such as those used to seal envelopes on holiday cards—to be sold at the Post Office for a penny each.

Bissell's campaign was endorsed by President Theodore Roosevelt and landed a feature in the *Philadelphia North American* newspaper. The surge of publicity helped Bissell's team of volunteers raise ten times their original modest goal of $300.

In 1908, Christmas Seals became a national campaign with a goal of advancing the fight against tuberculosis and providing support for sanatoriums all over the country. Millions of Christmas Seals were printed that year, raising $135,000—and thus, an annual holiday tradition began.

In 1920, the National Tuberculosis Association, which had previously been called the National Association for the Study and Prevention of Tuberculosis and would become the American Lung Association, took over the fundraising, employing a nationwide direct mailing campaign. Endorsed each year by celebrities and public figures, the Christmas Seals campaign became the first direct mail fundraiser focused on advancing the treatment of an infectious disease.

The American Lung Association's direct mail fundraising peaked around 1990, sending eighty million pieces of mail and raising $60,000,000 that year. Emily Bissell led the Christmas Seals campaign into the 1940s and was honored with her own commemorative postage stamp in 1980.

Question: **Was Bram Stoker's *Dracula* based on an infectious disease?**

Answer: The concept of vampires and vampirism existed before Bram Stoker's 1897 gothic horror novel *Dracula*. Superstitions about undead creatures existed throughout the Middle Ages as plague ravaged populations throughout Europe. It wasn't unusual to exhume bodies of the dead to examine them for signs of vampirism and to drive a stake through the heart of a body that was suspected of undead behavior.

Stoker's enigmatic and brooding Count Dracula may have been named for Vlad Dracula, also known as the brutal Vlad the Impaler, who was born in Transylvania, Romania, and ruled Walachia, Romania, intermittently between 1448 and 1476. Other details of Stoker's legendary vampire were taken from Slavic folktales.

Dracula eventually became the standard by which all other vampire myths are measured, but the first use of the word *vampire* in the English language seems to have occurred in newspaper articles in the 1730s. Rural European peasants reported incidences of unearthed bloodied and bloated corpses, contributing to the tales of the undead, who rose from the grave and subsisted on the blood of humans and animals.

Researchers have hypothesized that the mythology of vampires, as well as werewolves and zombies, may have stemmed from the symptoms and side effects of a number of illnesses and conditions, both genetic and infectious.

Infectious diseases such as rabies, syphilis, Zika virus, and bovine spongiform encephalopathy (mad cow disease) could have contributed to early myths and legends about vampires, werewolves, and zombies. But even in the era of modern medicine, novels and films often feature stories about incurable infectious pathogens.

Question: What is the "miracle toxin?"

Answer: One of the most poisonous known biological substances, botulinum toxin is a neurotoxin made by the common bacterium *Clostridium botulinum*. Botulinum toxin can cause botulism, a rare but dangerous condition that causes muscle weakness and paralysis and can lead to death.

Although botulinum toxin can lead to life-threatening illness, it also has medical and therapeutic uses, hence its nickname, the miracle toxin. When used in very small quantities, botulinum toxin is a muscle relaxant and is used as a treatment for some neuromuscular diseases. It can also be used as a cosmetic treatment for smoothing aging skin. The most widely known commercial form of botulinum toxin is marketed under the brand name Botox.

Seven types of botulinum toxin have been identified, and they are named from A to G. Occasionally, new types of the toxin are found. Types A and B are used in creating botulinum toxin injections for humans, with the botulinum toxin being purified and diluted with human serum albumin before use.

Question: What novels and movies feature plotlines about infectious diseases and pandemics?

Answer: The list of novels and movies about pathogens that cause everything from A (apocalypse) to Z (zombies) is lengthy. Some creative works center on fictional accounts of real infectious diseases, while others envision terrifying new viruses that wreak havoc on the world.

Some notable novels and films about infectious diseases and pandemics include these:

- *12 Monkeys* (1995 film)
- *28 Days Later* (2002 film)
- *The Andromeda Strain* by Michael Crichton (1969 novel, adapted for film in 1971)
- *Blindness* by José Saramago (1995 novel)
- *Contagion* (2011 film)
- *The Eyes of Darkness* by Dean Koontz (1981 novel)
- *The Host* (2006 film)
- *The Hot Zone: A Terrifying True Story* by Richard Preston (1994 nonfiction thriller)
- *I Am Legend* by Richard Matheson (1954 novel, adapted for film in 2007)
- *The Immune* by David Kazzie (2015 novel)
- *Outbreak* (1995 film, inspired by *The Hot Zone*)
- *The Plague* by Albert Camus (1947 novel)
- *The Seventh Seal* (1957 film)
- *The Stand* by Stephen King (1978 novel, adapted for television miniseries in 1994 and 2020)
- *Station Eleven* by Emily St. John Mandel (2014 novel)
- *World War Z* by Max Brooks (2006 novel, adapted for film in 2013)
- *Zone One* by Colson Whitehead (2011 novel)

Question: Why does the CDC have a zombie preparedness plan? Could a zombie apocalypse really happen?

Answer: The CDC's zombie preparedness plan doesn't actually have anything to do with zombies (which may be disappointing to some people). Zombies, like vampires and werewolves, have been a part of folklore for centuries. Pathogens, such as toxins found in animals like puffer fish, may have contributed to the mythology around zombies, with stories of people rising from the dead and behaving in uncharacteristic—and often cannibalistic—fashion. But although it may make for interesting conversation, a zombie apocalypse is just entertaining fiction.

In 2011, the CDC used the idea of a zombie apocalypse as a campaign to promote public awareness about the importance of being prepared for emergencies. "Preparedness 101: Zombie Apocalypse" was a blog post written by Rear Admiral Ali S. Khan, director of the CDC's Office of Public Health Preparedness and Response.

The campaign, based on the premise that being prepared for a zombie apocalypse would prepare you for any emergency, had three goals:

- To raise public awareness about emergency preparedness for the 2011 hurricane season
- To keep costs of the campaign low by using existing CDC resources and content
- To engage new audiences, particularly young people

Khan's tongue-in-cheek blog post succeeded on all counts. The first social media post on Twitter about the CDC's zombie preparedness plan generated so much internet traffic that it crashed the CDC website within ten minutes.

The popularity of "Preparedness 101: Zombie Apocalypse" led to posters, T-shirts, a graphic novella, and other zombie-themed activities and events.

Question: **Who were the first public figures to test positive for COVID-19? Have any famous people died of COVID-19?**

Answer: In the early months of the COVID-19 pandemic, dozens of celebrities, politicians, and other public figures took to social media or otherwise made announcements about having tested positive for the novel coronavirus.

On March 11, 2020, Academy Award–winning actor Tom Hanks and his wife, actress and musician Rita Wilson, became the first high-profile couple to announce they had tested positive for the virus. At the time, the pair were on location filming in Australia. The couple were quarantined and received treatment in Australia before returning to the United States two weeks later, where they continued to self-isolate and social distance. Hanks and Wilson made a full recovery from the illness.

These are other famous people who have announced that they'd contracted COVID-19:

- Albert II, Prince of Monaco
- Jackson Browne (singer-songwriter)
- Charles, Prince of Wales
- Chris Cuomo (CNN anchor)
- James Dolan (owner of the New York Knicks)

- Plácido Domingo (opera singer)
- Kevin Durant and several teammates (NBA player, Brooklyn Nets)
- Idris Elba (actor)
- Marianne Faithfull (singer-songwriter)
- Rudy Gobert and Donavan Mitchell (NBA players, Utah Jazz
- Boris Johnson (British prime minster)
- Daniel Dae Kim (actor)
- Rand Paul (US senator from Kentucky)
- Pink (singer-songwriter) and her three-year-old son
- Tony Shalhoub and his wife, Brooke Adams (actors)
- Lesley Stahl (*60 Minutes* journalist)
- George Stephanopoulos (political commentator) and his wife, Ali Wentworth (actor and writer)
- Sophie Grégoire Trudeau (wife of Canadian prime minister Justin Trudeau)
- Donald Trump (President of the United States) and his wife, Melania
- Prince William, Duke of Cambridge

Sadly, some public figures died in 2020 as a result of COVID-19. Among them were these people:

- Manu Dibango (saxophonist), died March 24
- Terrence McNally (playwright and screenwriter), died March 24
- Floyd Cardoz (celebrity chef), died March 25
- Joe Diffie (country music singer), died March 29

- Adam Schlesinger (singer-songwriter and cofounder of Fountains of Wayne), died April 1
- Ellis Marsalis Jr. (jazz musician and father of Wynton and Brandford), died April 1
- Tom Dempsey (former record-breaking NFL kicker), died April 4
- John Prine (singer-songwriter), died April 7
- Troy Sneed (gospel singer), died April 27
- Annie Glenn (widow of astronaut John Glenn), died May 19
- Nick Cordero (actor), died July 5
- Herman Cain (business executive, 2012 presidential candidate), died July 30
- Tom Seaver (Hall of Fame baseball player), died August 31

CHAPTER 10

HOW TO STAY HEALTHY

Wellness Myths, Home Remedies, Good Hygiene—And What You Should Do to Protect Yourself from Getting Sick

Question: What song should you sing to make sure you have thoroughly washed your hands?

Answer: Good handwashing hygiene is an important part of staying healthy and preventing the spread of disease. The World Health Organization provides a *handy* tutorial on how to wash your hands, emphasizing that the backs of the hands and the areas between the fingers need proper attention too. But knowing how long to wash is a little trickier.

The WHO's recommendation is that handwashing—the lathering and rubbing part—should last at least twenty seconds—or as long as it takes to sing (or hum) "Happy Birthday to You" twice.

Not a fan of "Happy Birthday to You"? That's okay. "The Alphabet Song" or "Row, Row, Row Your Boat" work too, or you can time yourself by singing the first chorus or two of your favorite song. Even better, Wash Your Lyrics (washyourlyrics.com) will customize your handwashing experience by generating a downloadable handwashing infographic to go along with your favorite song.

Question: Are there any home remedies that actually work to prevent a cold or the flu?

Answer: Most home remedies alleviate the symptoms of an illness and encourage a speedier recovery—but they don't necessarily prevent the illness itself.

Some home remedies, such as honey, as well as dietary supplements, such as vitamin D, may help alleviate symptoms, shorten the duration of an illness, or even reduce the chances of getting sick. But the best way to avoid the common cold or seasonal influenza is to wash your hands well and often and to avoid coming into contact with people who are sick. Reducing stress, getting enough rest, and staying hydrated are also important ways to maintain your health.

Question: **What is the difference between raw milk and milk that has been pasteurized?**

Answer: Raw milk is milk that comes directly from an animal and has not been altered in any way. This milk can carry bacteria that may cause foodborne illnesses.

Pasteurized milk is milk that has been heated to eliminate potentially harmful bacteria. Named for French scientist Louis Pasteur, who first experimented in the 1860s with heating wine and beer to prevent abnormal fermentation, there are different pasteurization processes used today to remove disease-causing pathogens and extend the shelf life of milk and other dairy products.

In the United States, most commercially produced milk is both pasteurized and homogenized. Homogenized milk is milk that has undergone a mechanical process to break down fat molecules in the milk in order to prevent separation and create a smooth, uniform consistency. Homogenization is not a safety process like pasteurization.

Question: Does chicken soup cure the common cold? And does it matter whether it's Grandma's homemade soup or store-bought?

Answer: As home remedies go, you could do worse than a bowl of homemade chicken soup. This soothing comfort food may actually offer some mild benefits when you're sick with a cold.

Research suggests that any warm liquid can help to clear nasal congestion and thin mucus for a more productive cough. But chicken soup in particular does a better job than other warm liquids because it improves the function of cilia, microscopic hairlike structures in the nose that help prevent contagions from entering the body.

And, in a study conducted in 2000 by Stephen Rennard, MD, of the University of Nebraska Medical Center, blood samples from volunteers showed that chicken soup inhibited the movement of neutrophils, the most common type of infection-fighting white blood cell. Rennard hypothesized that chicken soup aids in the reduction of upper-respiratory cold symptoms by working to limit the migration of neutrophils.

Rennard used his wife's chicken soup to conduct his research, a recipe handed down by her Lithuanian grandmother that called for an array of vegetables, including onions, carrots, and sweet potatoes. But research using commercial chicken soups yielded comparable results.

Question: What does "Feed a cold, starve a fever" mean—and does it work?

Answer: The adage "Feed a cold, starve a fever" dates back to at least 1574, when an English dictionary advised that fasting was beneficial in alleviating a fever.

Although illness can lead to a loss of appetite, eating nutritious food can give the body the energy to fight a cold virus. But starving a fever, which is the body's immune system response to fighting infection, may be counterintuitive. Fever elevates the body temperature, increasing the metabolism and burning calories at a faster pace—making calorie intake possibly just as important with a fever as with a cold.

However, staying hydrated during a fever is even more important than eating. So liquids, including soup, but excluding caffeine and alcohol, are particularly beneficial when suffering with a fever.

Other research suggests that it's less about whether you have a cold or fever than it is about the cause of your illness. Studies indicate that eating can produce the immune response necessary for combating a viral infection, such as a cold, while fasting may result in an immune response that works against a bacterial infection. Because a fever can be the result of either a virus or bacteria, knowing the source of the fever may be helpful in knowing whether to "starve" that fever.

Question: Do bedbugs transmit infectious diseases?

Answer: The saying "Good night, sleep tight, don't let the bedbugs bite" might seem to refer to the insects as disease vectors, but this is one bug that isn't known to transmit illness.

Bedbugs are nuisance pests that feast on human blood and can be found where people sleep. These insects live in all parts of the world and are not an indicator of cleanliness, or a lack thereof. But bedbugs can cause itching, which could lead to excessive scratching and an increased risk of a secondary skin infection.

Question: What is the best way to protect yourself against an infectious disease?

Answer: For healthy people with no underlying illness, the simplest way to prevent infection is to practice good personal hygiene. Good hygiene not only helps prevent infection, it also works to help prevent the spread of infection.

Good personal hygiene habits include the following:

- Washing your hands thoroughly
  - before preparing or eating food.
  - after using the bathroom.
  - after coughing, sneezing, or blowing your nose.
  - after gardening or other outdoor tasks.

- after feeding, touching, or playing with your pet or other animal.
- before and after visiting or caring for a sick person.

- Covering your cough or sneeze
  - Cough or sneeze into a tissue and dispose of the tissue immediately.
  - If you don't have a tissue, cough or sneeze into your elbow instead of your hand.

- Taking care of wounds
  - Wash and bandage all cuts, and do not pick at healing wounds or blemishes.
  - Have animal or human bites and serious cuts examined by a doctor.

- Avoiding sharing dishes, eating utensils, glasses, water bottles, or straws
  - This is particularly important with people outside your household.

- Avoiding direct contact with tissues, napkins, and other similar items used by other people

Question: Is it true that "Ring around the Rosie" was about the Black Death?

Answer: Urban legend holds that the childhood nursery rhyme "Ring around the Rosie" (or other versions, such as the British "Ring-a-ring o' Roses") references the horrors of the Black Death in England during the fourteenth century. One of the most popular versions of the rhyme is as follows:

> *Ring around the rosie,*
>
> *Pocket full of posies,*
>
> *Ashes, ashes*
>
> *We all fall down!*

It's not known when the nursery rhyme was written, but printed appearances date to the mid- to late-nineteenth century, with Kate Greenaway's 1881 *Mother Goose or the Old Nursery Rhymes* being a well-known early appearance of the rhyme.

Although many variations of the nursery rhyme have circulated in different parts of the world, the lack of documentation prior to the 1800s makes it unlikely that "Ring around the Rosie" references an event that happened five hundred years earlier. In fact, the plague interpretation of the rhyme seems to have begun circulating in the mid-twentieth century. Today most folklorists agree that the rhyme has no definitive origin or meaning.

Question: **Why do some countries require pets from foreign countries be quarantined upon entry?**

Answer: Some countries, many of them island nations, do not have diseases that are found in other parts of the world, such as rabies. As a result, these countries have strict policies to make sure a new disease isn't introduced into their country.

In addition to proof of rabies vaccination, some countries require that a pet be quarantined upon entry to ensure they are disease-free. These are some of the countries with pet quarantines:

- Australia
- Fiji
- Guam
- Hong Kong
- Iceland
- Japan
- Malaysia
- New Zealand
- Singapore
- Taiwan

In the United States, Hawaii also has a quarantine for pets because the island state is rabies-free.

Guidelines in all countries are subject to change based on several factors, including the prevalence of rabies in a pet's country of origin. Because dog rabies was eliminated in the United States in 2007, the guidelines about entering the United States focus on avoiding importing dog rabies from high-risk countries.

Question: **What is tetanus, and why are we always being told to get a tetanus shot?**

Answer: If you have ever stepped on a rusty nail or cut yourself on a chain-link fence, someone probably asked, "Have you had a tetanus shot?"

Tetanus is an acute infectious disease caused by bacteria spores in the environment. The spores of the bacterium *Clostridium tetani* that cause tetanus can be found almost everywhere, including in soil, in animal and human feces, on the surface of the skin, and on rusty metal, such as nails and barbed wire. The bacteria spores are resistant to heat and to most antiseptics and therefore can survive for a long time—even years.

Tetanus is also called lockjaw because a common sign of a tetanus infection is the tightening of the jaw muscles, which causes cramping or even the inability to open the mouth. Other symptoms of tetanus include the following:

- Changes in blood pressure
- Difficulty swallowing
- Fever and sweating
- Headache
- Muscle spasms, most often in the back, stomach, arms, and legs
- Muscle spasms triggered by sudden noises
- Rapid heart rate
- Seizures

Immunization with tetanus-toxoid-containing vaccines (TTCV) can prevent tetanus. To be fully protected for life, the World Health Organization recommends six doses—three primary and three boosters—of TTCV. The primary series of TTCV immunizations can start as early as six weeks after birth, with spaced intervals recommended for both the primary and booster doses.

Although anyone can get tetanus, those most at risk include pregnant women who have not been immunized and newborn babies. For that reason, tetanus is of particular concern in low-income communities and countries where immunization rates are low and birth practices may be unclean.

The first tetanus-toxoid vaccine was introduced in the United States in the late 1940s. Today, tetanus is rare in the United States, with only around thirty cases reported each year—most often in people who were never given a tetanus vaccine or who did not complete the recommended course of tetanus vaccines, or adults who haven't stayed up to date on the recommended booster vaccines. Staying current on recommended booster vaccinations and practicing good wound care are the best ways to prevent tetanus.

Protection against tetanus and diphtheria, and often whooping cough (pertussis) is administered as a single vaccine. Infants and children younger than seven receive DTaP (or DT) vaccines, while older children and adults receive Tdap (or Td) vaccines. In the United States, the CDC recommends adults receive a Tdap or Td shot every ten years.

Question: How does deforestation contribute to the increase of infectious diseases?

Answer: Research has shown that deforestation—the cutting down of large areas of forested land—can lead to a rise in infectious diseases.

Around 60 percent of the viruses that affect humans begin as zoonotic viruses in animals, both domestic and wild. Deforestation creates an environment in which disease can thrive, and the greater the number of animal and insect species that are affected by deforestation in a particular area, the greater the number of diseases that can affect humans.

Research has documented a spike in infectious diseases, such as malaria and dengue, as a result of deforestation. Scientists are concerned about an increased risk of a global pandemic as a result of the ecological disturbances caused by deforestation.

Question: **Can you catch an infectious disease from touching a surface (such as in a public restroom) that has been contaminated by a virus?**

Answer: The short answer is no, it is virtually impossible for a person to become sick from touching a surface contaminated by a virus.

Viruses that cause infectious diseases thrive in the body—but once expelled, either in bodily fluids or through breathing, coughing, or sneezing, many viruses can continue to live outside the host body. But how long a particular virus lives outside the body depends on several conditions, including temperature and level of moisture. Some viruses can live longer on water-resistant, nonporous surfaces, such as plastic or stainless steel.

But although many disease-causing organisms can live for a short while on hard surfaces, such as a door handle or toilet seat, a healthy immune system, along with good handwashing hygiene, is usually enough to protect most people from illness.

For an infection to occur, germs would have to be transferred from the surface of a door handle or toilet seat and introduced into the body, either through the mouth, nose, eyes, urethral tract, or genital tract, or through an open cut or sore.

BIBLIOGRAPHY AND FURTHER READING

"8 Zoonotic Diseases Shared Between Animals and People of Most Concern in the U.S." *CDC.gov*. Last modified May 6, 2019. https://www.cdc.gov/media/releases/2019/s0506-zoonotic-diseases-shared.html.

"The 9 Deadly Diseases That Plagued George Washington." *PBS.org*. July 4, 2011. https://www.pbs.org/newshour/health/george-washingtons-medical-chart.

"14 Diseases You Almost Forgot About (Thanks to Vaccines)." *CDC.gov*. Last modified January 3, 2020. https://www.cdc.gov/vaccines/parents/diseases/forgot-14-diseases.html.

"1908 American Red Cross Christmas Seal—Type I, Perf 14, Smooth Gum." *Mysticstamp.com*. Accessed August 2, 2020. https://www.mysticstamp.com/Products/United-States/WX3/USA.

"The 1918 Flu Pandemic: Why It Matters 100 Years Later." *CDC.gov*. Last modified May 14, 2018. https://blogs.cdc.gov/publichealthmatters/2018/05/1918-flu.

"2009 H1N1 Pandemic (H1N1pdm09 Virus)." *CDC.gov*. Last modified June 11, 2019. https://www.cdc.gov/flu/pandemic-resources/2009-h1n1-pandemic.html.

"2019–2020 U.S. Flu Season: Preliminary Burden Estimates." *CDC.gov*. Last modified April 17, 2020. https://www.cdc.gov/flu/about/burden/preliminary-in-season-estimates.htm.

"37th Anniversary of the First Reported Cases of AIDS in the United States." *HIV.gov*. June 5, 2018. https://www.hiv.gov/blog/37th-anniversary-first-reported-cases-aids-united-states.

"About the NIH." *NIH.gov*. July 7, 2015. https://www.nih.gov/about-nih/what-we-do/nih-almanac/about-nih.

"About Quarantine and Isolation." *CDC.gov*. Last modified January 27, 2020. https://www.cdc.gov/quarantine/quarantineisolation.html.

Ainsworth, Claire, and Damian Carrington. "BSE Disaster: The History." *New Scientist*, October 25, 2000. https://www.newscientist.com/article/dn91-bse-disaster-the-history.

"All About BSE (Mad Cow Disease)." *FDA.gov*. Last modified July 23, 2020. https://www.fda.gov/animal-veterinary/animal-health-literacy/all-about-bse-mad-cow-disease.

"The American Lung Association." *Postalmuseum.si.edu*. Accessed August 7, 2020. https://postalmuseum.si.edu/exhibition/america's-mailing-industry-industry-segments-nonprofit-organizations/the-american-lung.

Andrews, Evan. "Why Was It Called the 'Spanish Flu'?" *History.com*. Last updated March 27, 2020. https://www.history.com/news/why-was-it-called-the-spanish-flu.

Arguelles, Juan-Carlos. "The Early Days of the Nobel Prize and Golden Age of Microbiology." *Hektoen International*. Last modified February 1, 2017. https://hekint.org/2017/02/01/the-early-days-of-the-nobel-prize-and-golden-age-of-microbiology/.

Aryal, Sagar. "Epidemic—Causes, Types, and Response: Epidemiology." *Microbenotes.com*, January 11, 2020. https://microbenotes.com/epidemic-causes-types-and-response.

Ault, Alicia. "Ask Smithsonian: Is the World Due for Another Massive Plague Outbreak?" *Smithsonian*, October 22, 2015. https://www.smithsonianmag.com/smithsonian-institution/ask-smithsonian-world-due-another-massive-plague-outbreak-180957001.

Baicus, Anda. "History of Polio Vaccination." *World Journal of Virology* 1, no. 4 (August 2012): 108–14. https://www.ncbi.nlm.nih.gov/pmc/articles/PMC3782271.

Barbash, Fred. "Here's to George Washington, Afflicted with So Many Killer Diseases It's Miraculous He Survived to Become Father of Our Nation." *Washington Post*, February 22, 2017. https://www.washingtonpost.com/news/morning-mix/wp/2017/02/22/heres-to-george-washington-afflicted-with-so-many-killer-diseases-its-miraculous-he-became-father-of-our-nation.

Barberis, I., P. Myles, S. K. Ault, N. L. Bragazzi, and M. Martini. "History and Evolution of Influenza Control Through Vaccination: From the First Monovalent Vaccine to Universal Vaccines." *Journal of Preventive Medicine and Hygiene* 57, no. 3 (2016): E115–E120. https://www.ncbi.nlm.nih.gov/pmc/articles/PMC5139605.

Barrett, Michael. "How a Generation of Consumptives Defined 19th-Century Romanticism." *Aeon*, April 10, 2017. https://aeon.co/ideas/how-a-generation-of-consumptives-defined-19th-century-romanticism.

Barry, John M. *The Great Influenza: The Story of the Deadliest Pandemic in History*. New York: Viking Press, 2004.

"Vaccines: The Basics." *CDC.gov*. Last modified March 14, 2012. https://www.cdc.gov/vaccines/vpd/vpd-vac-basics.html.

Bates Ramirez, Vanessa. "What Is R0? Gauging Contagious Infections." *Healthline*, April 20, 2020. https://www.healthline.com/health/r-nought-reproduction-number.

"Bed Bugs—Frequently Asked Questions (FAQs)." *CDC.gov*. Last modified January 4, 2017. https://www.cdc.gov/parasites/bedbugs/faqs.html.

Bergman, Rachel. "CDC: Fewer than Half of Americans Get Flu Vaccine." *The Nation's Health*, November 1, 2017. https://thenationshealth.aphapublications.org/content/47/9/E45.

"Biological Weapons." *WHO.int*. Last modified August 3, 2020. https://www.who.int/health-topics/biological-weapons.

"The Biological Weapons Convention (BWC) at a Glance." *Armscontrol.gov*. Last modified March 2020. https://www.armscontrol.org/factsheets/bwc.

"Bioterrorism Agents/Diseases." *CDC.gov*. Last modified April 4, 2018. https://emergency.cdc.gov/agent/agentlist-category.asp.

Blakemore, Erin. "Why Plague Doctors Wore Those Strange Beaked Masks." *National Geographic*, March 12, 2020. https://www.nationalgeographic.com/history/reference/european-history/plague-doctors-beaked-masks-coronavirus.

Board of Governors of the Federal Reserve System. *FederalReserve.gov*. Last modified August 7, 2020. https://www.federalreserve.gov/faqs/why-do-us-coins-seem-to-be-in-short-supply-coin-shortage.htm.

Bolinger, Hope. "Who Are the Four Horsemen in Revelation? Their Meaning and Significance." *Christianity.com*, May 21, 2019. https://www.christianity.com/wiki/end-times/who-are-the-four-horsemen-in-revelation-their-meaning-and-significance.html.

Bradley, Jeanette. "These 4 Vaccines May Pose a Risk If You're Allergic to Eggs." *Verywell Health*. Last modified November 27, 2019. https://www.verywellhealth.com/can-you-get-vaccines-if-you-are-allergic-to-eggs-1324082.

Branswell, Helen. "The New Pneumonia-Causing Virus Needs a Name. It May Be Tricky." *Stat*, January 23, 2020. https://www.statnews.com/2020/01/23/its-been-sequenced-its-spread-across-borders-now-the-new-pneumonia-causing-virus-needs-a-name.

Broom, Douglas. "5 Charts That Tell the Story of Vaccines Today." *World Economic Forum*. June 2, 2020. https://www.weforum.org/agenda/2020/06/vaccine-development-barriers-coronavirus.

"Brucellosis." *CDC.gov*. Last modified March 8, 2019. https://www.cdc.gov/brucellosis/index.html.

Bruzek, Alison. "Ebola in the United States: What Happened When." *NPR*, October 15, 2014. https://www.npr.org/sections/health-shots/2014/10/15/356098903/ebola-in-the-united-states-what-happened-when.

Bulit, David. "A. G. Holley State Tuberculosis Hospital." *Abandoned Florida*, June 28, 2020. https://www.abandonedfl.com/a-g-holley-state-hospital.

Bush, Larry M., and Maria T. Vazquez-Pertejo. "Botulism—Infectious Diseases." *Merck Manual*. Last modified September 2019. https://www.merckmanuals.com/professional/infectious-diseases/anaerobic-bacteria/botulism.

Caceres, Vanessa. "What's the Difference Between an Epidemic and Pandemic?" *U.S. News & World Report*, March 13, 2020. https://health.usnews.com/conditions/articles/whats-the-difference-between-an-epidemic-and-pandemic.

Calderone, Julia. "Christopher Columbus Brought a Host of Terrible New Diseases to the New World." *Business Insider*, October 12, 2015. https://www.businessinsider.com/diseases-columbus-brought-to-americas-2015-10.

Campbell, Charlie, and Alice Park. "Where Did Coronavirus Originate? Inside the Hunt to Find Out." *Time*, July 23, 2020. https://time.com/5870481/coronavirus-origins/.

"CDC: The Nation's Prevention Agency." *CDC.gov*. Last modified August 25, 2020. https://www.cdc.gov/mmwr/preview/mmwrhtml/00017924.htm.

"CDC's Zombie Preparedness—A Great Example of Edutainment IMC." *Letstalkpublichealth.com*, December 10, 2017. https://www.letstalk publichealth.com/blog/cdc-zombie-preparedness-edutainment.

Center for Devices and Radiological Health. "N95 Respirators, Surgical Masks, and Face Masks." US Food and Drug Administration. *FDA.gov*. Last modified August 2020. https://www.fda.gov/medical-devices /personal-protective-equipment-infection-control/n95-respirators -surgical-masks-and-face-masks.

Chan-Tack, Kirk M. "Botulism Clinical Presentation: History, Physical, Causes." *Medscape*. Last modified February 15, 2019. https:// emedicine.medscape.com/article/213311-clinical.

Chang, Bettina. "'House' Fans Are Scared of the Wrong Diseases." *Pacific Standard*. Last modified June 14, 2017. https://psmag.com /social-justice/house-fans-scared-wrong-diseases-84783.

Chen, Angus. "Why Haven't We Cured the Common Cold Yet?" *Scientific American,* September 4, 2018. https://www.scientific american.com/article/why-havent-we-cured-the-common -cold-yet/.

Chen, Caroline. "What We Need to Understand About Asymptomatic Carriers If We're Going to Beat Coronavirus." *ProPublica*, April 2, 2020. https://www.propublica.org/article/what-we-need-to-understand -about-asymptomatic-carriers-if-were-going-to-beat- coronavirus.

Cheng, Vincent C. C., Susanna K. P. Lau, Patrick C. Y. Woo, and Kwok Yung Yuen. "Severe Acute Respiratory Syndrome Coronavirus as an Agent of Emerging and Reemerging Infection." *Clinical Microbiology Reviews* 20, no. 4 (2007): 660–64. https://cmr.asm.org/content/20 /4/660.

Chotiner, Isaac. "How Pandemics Change History." *The New Yorker*, March 3, 2020. https://www.newyorker.com/news/q-and-a/how -pandemics-change-history.

Clarke, Imogen. "Tuberculosis: A Fashionable Disease?" *Science Museum Blog*, March 24, 2019. https://blog.sciencemuseum.org.uk /tuberculosis-a-fashionable-disease/.

"Clean Hands Protect Against Infection." *World Health Organization*. Last modified June 8, 2011. https://www.who.int/teams/integrated -health-services/infection-prevention-control.

"Cold Versus Flu." *CDC.gov*. Last modified December 30, 2019. https://www.cdc.gov/flu/symptoms/coldflu.htm.

Collis, Clark. "'Our Pitch Was, It's Going to Be Scary': Inside the Making of Lockdown Horror Movie 'Host.'" *EW.com*, August 17, 2020. https://ew.com/movies/host-lockdown-horror-movie-rob-savage/.

"The Continuum of Pandemic Phases." *CDC.gov*. Last modified November 3, 2016. https://www.cdc.gov/flu/pandemic-resources/planning-preparedness/global-planning-508.html.

Cooper, Laura, Su Yun Kang, Donal Bisanzio, Kilama Maxwell, Isabel Rodriguez-Barraquer, Bryan Greenhouse, Chris Drakeley et al. "Pareto Rules for Malaria Super-Spreaders and Super-Spreading." *Nature* 10, no. 3939 (2019). https://www.nature.com/articles/s41467-019-11861-y.

"Coronavirus." *CDC.gov*. Last modified February 15, 2020. https://www.cdc.gov/coronavirus/types.html.

"Coronavirus (Covid-19) Frequently Asked Questions." *CDC.gov*. Last modified November 13, 2020. https://www.cdc.gov/coronavirus/2019-ncov/faq.html.

Corona, Angel. "Disease Eradication: What Does It Take to Wipe Out a Disease?" *ASM.org*, March 6, 2020. https://asm.org/Articles/2020/March/Disease-Eradication-What-Does-It-Take-to-Wipe-out.

"Coronavirus Disease 2019 (Covid-19)." *CDC.gov*. Last modified August 15, 2020. https://www.cdc.gov/coronavirus/2019-ncov/index.html.

Cox, Joanne E., and Tina L. Cheng. "Egg-Based Vaccines." *American Academy of Pediatrics* 27, no. 3 (2006): 118–19. https://pedsinreview.aappublications.org/content/27/3/118.

Cuncic, Arlin. "Many People with Depression Also Have Comorbidity." *Verywellmind.com*, March 27, 2020. https://www.verywellmind.com/what-is-comorbidity-3024480.

Cunha, Burke A. "The Death of Alexander the Great: Malaria or Typhoid Fever?" *Infectious Disease Clinics of North America* 18, no. 1 (2004): 53–63. https://pubmed.ncbi.nlm.nih.gov/15081504/.

Day, Carolyn A. *Consumptive Chic: A History of Beauty, Fashion, and Disease*. London: Bloomsbury, 2020.

"The Deadly Virus." *National Archives and Records Administration.* Accessed June 25, 2020. https://www.archives.gov/exhibits/influenza-epidemic/records-list.html.

DerSarkissian, Carol. "Flu Vaccine Effectiveness: How Well Does It Work?" *WebMD.com.* Last modified August 26, 2019. https://www.webmd.com/vaccines/how-effective-is-flu-vaccine.

Diamond, Jared M. *Guns, Germs, and Steel: The Fates of Human Societies.* New York: W. W. Norton & Co., 1997.

"Disease Considered as Candidates for Global Eradication by the International Task Force for Disease Eradication." *Cartercenter.org,* 2008. https://www.cartercenter.org/resources/pdfs/news/health_publications/itfde/updated_disease_candidate_table.pdf.

Domonoske, Camila. "Whaddaya Knead? Yeast and Baking Powder Top America's Shopping Lists." *NPR,* April 3, 2020. https://www.npr.org/2020/04/03/826939405/whaddaya-knead-yeast-and-baking-powder-top-americas-shopping-lists.

Doucleff, Michaeleen. "Are There Zombie Viruses in the Thawing Permafrost?" *NPR,* January 24, 2018. https://www.npr.org/sections/goatsandsoda/2018/01/24/575974220/are-there-zombie-viruses-in-the-thawing-permafrost.

Dowling, Stephen. "The Real-Life Diseases That Spread the Vampire Myth." *BBC,* October 31, 2016. https://www.bbc.com/future/article/20161031-the-real-life-disease-that-spread-the-vampire-myth.

"Dr. Gerhard Armauer Hansen." *LeprosyHistory.org.* Accessed August 5, 2020. https://leprosyhistory.org/database/person1.

Dubos, René, and Jean Dubos. *The White Plague: Tuberculosis, Man and Society.* New Brunswick: Rutgers University Press, 1996.

"Ebola Virus Disease." *OIE: World Organization for Animal Health.* Last modified December 6, 2018. https://www.oie.int/en/animal-health-in-the-world/animal-diseases/ebola-virus-disease/.

Editorial Board. "Call It 'Coronavirus.'" *The New York Times,* March 23, 2020. https://www.nytimes.com/2020/03/23/opinion/china-coronavirus-racism.html.

Ehrenkranz, N. Joel, and Deborah A Sampson. "Origin of the Old Testament Plagues: Explications and Implications." *The Yale Journal of Biology and Medicine* 81, no. 1 (2008): 31–42. https://www.ncbi.nlm.nih.gov/pmc/articles/PMC2442724/.

"Fact Sheet: Explaining Operation Warp Speed." *HHS.gov*. Last modified October 14, 2020. https://www.hhs.gov/about/news/2020/06/16/fact-sheet-explaining-operation-warp-speed.html.

Fetters, Ashley. "From Haight Street to Sesame Street: The Evolution of AIDS in Pop Culture." *The Atlantic*, December 4, 2012. https://www.theatlantic.com/entertainment/archive/2012/12/from-haight-street-to-sesame-street-the-evolution-of-aids-in-pop-culture/265872/.

Firimbi, Piga. "The Troubled Suspected Covid-19 Intermediary Host." *PulitzerCenter.org*, August 12, 2020. https://pulitzercenter.org/reporting/troubled-suspected-Covid-19-intermediary-host.

Fischetti, Mark. "Fact or Fiction?: Feed a Cold, Starve a Fever." *Scientific American*, January 3, 2014. https://www.scientificamerican.com/article/fact-or-fiction-feed-a-cold.

Fisher, Max. "R0, The Messy Metric That May Soon Shape Our Lives, Explained." *The New York Times*, April 23, 2020. https://www.nytimes.com/2020/04/23/world/europe/coronavirus-R0-explainer.html.

Fleury, Bruce E. "Biological Warfare: The Geneva Protocol of 1925." *TheGreatCoursesDaily.com*, December 1, 2017. https://www.thegreatcoursesdaily.com/biological-warfare-the-geneva-protocol.

Fliesler, Nancy. "How Fast Can We Get a COVID-19 Vaccine?" *ChildrensHospital.org*. Last modified June 12, 2020. https://discoveries.childrenshospital.org/covid-19-vaccine.

"Flu Shot: Your Best Bet for Avoiding Influenza." *Mayo Clinic*. Last modified November 13, 2020. https://www.mayoclinic.org/diseases-conditions/flu/in-depth/flu-shots/art-20048000.

"Flu Vaccination Coverage, United States, 2018–19 Influenza Season." *CDC.gov*. Last modified September 26, 2019. https://www.cdc.gov/flu/fluvaxview/coverage-1819estimates.htm.

"Frequently Asked Questions and Answers on Smallpox." *World Health Organization*. Last modified June 28, 2016. https://www.who.int/csr/disease/smallpox/faq/en.

Frischknecht, Friedrich. "The History of Biological Warfare. Human Experimentation, Modern Nightmares and Lone Madmen in the Twentieth Century." *EMBO Reports* 4, no. 1 (2003): S47–S52. https://www.ncbi.nlm.nih.gov/pmc/articles/PMC1326439.

Frith, John. "The History of Plague—Part 1. The Three Great Pandemics." *Journal of Military and Veterans' Health* 20, no. 2 (2012). https://jmvh.org/article/the-history-of-plague-part-1-the-three-great-pandemics.

Gallagher, James. "Aids: Origin of Pandemic 'Was 1920s Kinshasa.'" *BBC News*, October 2, 2014. https://www.bbc.com/news/health-29442642.

Gander, Kashmira. "Smallpox Was Eradicated 40 Years Ago, So Why Are the U.S. and Russia Still Holding Stocks of the Virus?" *Newsweek*, December 13, 2019. https://www.newsweek.com/smallpox-eradicated-40-years-ago-us-russia-stocks-virus-1476932.

"The Germ Theory of Disease." *Prezi.com*. Accessed August 3, 2020. https://prezi.com/-crarn19mpig/the-germ-theory-of-disease.

Gillespie, Claire. "This Is How Many People Die from the Flu Each Year." *Health.com*. Last updated September 24, 2020. https://www.health.com/condition/cold-flu-sinus/how-many-people-die-of-the-flu-every-year.

"The Global HIV/AIDS Epidemic." *KFF.org*, July 13, 2020. https://www.kff.org/global-health-policy/fact-sheet/the-global-hivaids-epidemic/.

"Global HIV and AIDS Statistics—2020 Fact Sheet." *UNAIDS.org*. Accessed August 7, 2020. https://www.unaids.org/en/resources/fact-sheet.

Godoy, Maria. "A User's Guide to Masks: What's Best at Protecting Others (and Yourself)." *NPR*, July 1, 2020. https://www.npr.org/sections/goatsandsoda/2020/07/01/880621610/a-users-guide-to-masks-what-s-best-at-protecting-others-and-yourself.

Goldman, Rena, and Stephanie Watson. "Cold or Flu? How to Know Which One You Have." *Healthline*. Last modified September 9, 2020. https://www.healthline.com/health/cold-flu/cold-or-flu.

Gould, S. E. "Ancient Diseases of Human Ancestors." *Scientific American*, May 12, 2012. https://blogs.scientificamerican.com/lab-rat/ancient-diseases-of-human-ancestors/.

"Grandma's Chicken Soup." *Prevention.com*, March 12, 2016. https://www.prevention.com/food-nutrition/recipes/a20531505/grandmas-chicken-soup.

Griffiths, Sian, and Xiao-Nong Zhou. "Chapter 1: Why Research Infectious Diseases of Poverty?" Geneva: *World Health Organization*, 2012. https://www.who.int/tdr/stewardship/global_report/2012/chapitre1_web.pdf.

Groth, Leah. "Anthony Fauci's Baseball Card Broke a Sales Record." *Yahoo!*, July 30, 2020. https://www.yahoo.com/lifestyle/anthony-fauci-baseball-card-broke-055221579.html.

"Guns, Germs and Steel: Variables; Smallpox." *PBS*. Accessed August 13, 2020. https://www.pbs.org/gunsgermssteel/variables/smallpox.html.

Hartwyk, Cait. "What Killed Alexander the Great?" *PassportHealth.com,* June 20, 2017. https://www.passporthealthusa.com/2017/06/what-killed-alexander-the-great/.

"Herd Immunity and Covid-19 (Coronavirus): What You Need to Know." *Mayo Clinic*, June 6, 2020. https://www.mayoclinic.org/diseases-conditions/coronavirus/in-depth/herd-immunity-and-coronavirus/art-20486808.

Hewings-Martin, Yella. "How Do SARS and MERS Compare with COVID-19?" *MedicalNewsToday.com*, April 10, 2020. https://www.medicalnewstoday.com/articles/how-do-sars-and-mers-compare-with-covid-19.

Hickok, Kimberly. "Who Created the Polio Vaccine?" *LiveScience.com*, June 1, 2020. https://www.livescience.com/polio-virus-vaccine.html.

"History of AIDS." *History.com*. Last updated November 3, 2020. https://www.history.com/topics/1980s/history-of-aids.

"A History of Biological Weapons." *PBS*. Accessed August 6, 2020. https://www.pbs.org/wgbh/americanexperience/features/weapon-timeline.

"The History of Christmas Seals." *American Lung Association*. Accessed August 7, 2020. https://ala-web-staging-mvc-app.azurewebsites.net/get-involved/ways-to-give/christmas-seals/history.

"History of Quarantine." *CDC.gov*. Last modified July 20, 2020. https://www.cdc.gov/quarantine/historyquarantine.html.

"History of Vaccines Timeline." *History of Vaccines.org*. Accessed August 12, 2020. https://www.historyofvaccines.org/timeline/all.

"HIV/AIDS." *Mayo Clinic*, February 13, 2020. https://www.mayoclinic.org/diseases-conditions/hiv-aids/diagnosis-treatment/drc-20373531.

"HIV in the United States and Dependent Areas." *CDC.gov*. Last modified June 10, 2020. https://www.cdc.gov/hiv/statistics/overview/ataglance.html.

"How the Virus That Causes Covid-19 Differs from Other Coronaviruses." *NewsNetwork.com*. March 30, 2020. https://newsnetwork.mayoclinic.org/discussion/how-the-virus-that-causes-Covid-19-differs-from-other-coronaviruses/.

"How to Prevent Infections." *Harvard.edu*, August 2016. https://www.health.harvard.edu/staying-healthy/how-to-prevent-infections.

Hui, Mary. "Rt: The Number That Can Guide How Societies Ease Coronavirus Lockdowns." *Quartz*, April 8, 2020. https://qz.com/1834700/rt-the-real-time-r0-guiding-how-to-lift-coronavirus-lockdowns.

"How the Flu Virus Can Change: 'Drift' and 'Shift.'" *CDC.gov*. Last modified October 15, 2019. https://www.cdc.gov/flu/about/viruses/change.htm.

Hsu, Jeremy. "Germs on the Big Screen: 11 Infectious Movies." *LiveScience.com*, September 9, 2011. https://www.livescience.com/15982-infectious-disease-movies.html.

"Immunization Schedules." *CDC.gov*. Last modified February 3, 2020. https://www.cdc.gov/vaccines/schedules/index.html.

"Infectious Diseases." *Mayo Clinic*. Last modified July 17, 2019. https://www.mayoclinic.org/diseases-conditions/infectious-diseases/symptoms-causes/syc-20351173.

Infectious Diseases of Poverty. *Biomedcentral.com*. Accessed July 31, 2020. https://idpjournal.biomedcentral.com/.

"Influenza Historic Timeline." *CDC.gov*. Last modified January 30, 2019. https://www.cdc.gov/flu/pandemic-resources/pandemic-timeline-1930-and-beyond.htm.

"Influenza in Animals." *CDC.gov*. Last modified September 27, 2018. https://www.cdc.gov/flu/other/index.html.

"Introduction to Public Health Surveillance|Public Health 101 Series|CDC." *CDC.gov*. Last modified November 15, 2018. https://www.cdc.gov/publichealth101/surveillance.html.

Johnson, Eric Michael. "A Natural History of Vampires." *Scientific American.com*, October 31, 2011. https://blogs.scientificamerican .com/primate-diaries/a-natural-history-of-vampires.

Kawash, Samira. "The Candy Prophylactic: Danger, Disease, and Children's Candy Around 1916." *CandyProfessor.com*, September 8, 2010. https://candyprofessor.com/candy-bibliography-library /polio-and-childrens-candy-around-1916.

Kelly, John. *The Great Mortality: An Intimate History of the Black Death, the Most Devastating Plague of All Time.* New York: HarperCollins, 2005.

"Keyword Search: Pestilence." *BibleGateway.com*. Accessed August 4, 2020. https://www.biblegateway.com/quicksearch/?quicksearch =pestilence.

"Keyword Search: Plague." *BibleGateway.com*. Accessed August 4, 2020. https://www.biblegateway.com/quicksearch/?quicksearch =plague.

Khamsi, Roxanne. "Were 'Cursed' Rams the First Biological Weapons?" *NewScientist*, November 26, 2007. https://www.new scientist.com/article/dn12960-were-cursed-rams-the-first -biological-weapons.

Kinch, Michael S. "What a Sugar Cube Can Teach Us as We Develop a Coronavirus Vaccine." *CNN*, April 23, 2020. https://www.cnn.com /2020/04/23/opinions/polio-sugar-cube-coronavirus-vaccine -kinch/index.html.

"Kinds of Botulism." *CDC.gov*. Last modified August 19, 2019. https://www.cdc.gov/botulism/definition.html.

Koenig, Debbie. "2019 Measles Outbreak: What You Should Know." *WebMD.com*, April 11, 2019. https://www.webmd.com/children /news/20190411/2019-measles-outbreak-what-you-should-know.

Kolata, Gina. "How Pandemics End." *The New York Times*. Last modified May 14, 2020. https://www.nytimes.com/2020/05/10 /health/coronavirus-plague-pandemic-history.html.

Kravitz, Melissa. "What to Do If You Get Sick While Traveling—and How to Stay Healthy Before You Leave (video)." *TravelandLeisure.com*, February 14, 2020. https://www.travelandleisure.com/travel-tips /what-to-do-sick-when-traveling.

Kritz, Fran. "Russian Lab Explosion Raises Question: Should Smallpox Virus Be Kept or Destroyed?" *NPR*, September 19, 2019. https://www.npr.org/sections/goatsandsoda/2019/09/19/762013515/russian-lab-explosion-raises-question-should-smallpox-virus-be-kept-or-destroyed.

Kruse, Kevin. "The 80/20 Rule and How It Can Change Your Life." *Forbes*. Last modified March 7, 2016. https://www.forbes.com/sites/kevinkruse/2016/03/07/80-20-rule.

Kucharski, Adam. *The Rules of Contagion: Why Things Spread and Why They Stop*. New York: Basic Books, 2020.

Lall, Kriti. "To Destroy or to Not Destroy?" *Nature*, January 26, 2015. https://www.nature.com/scitable/blog/microbe-matters/to_destroy_or_to_not/.

Lam, Jerika, and Jeff Goad. "The Burden of Vaccine-Preventable Diseases in Adults." *PharmacyTimes.com*, March 31, 2017. https://www.pharmacytimes.com/publications/supplementals/2017/immunizationsupplementmarch2017/the-burden-of-vaccine preventable-diseases-in-adults.

Larson, Jennifer. "When Is Flu Season and Why There Is a Flu Season in the First Place." *Insider*. Last modified May 1, 2020. https://www.insider.com/when-is-flu-season.

Lava, Neil. "Mad Cow Disease: Symptoms, Causes and Treatments for VCJD." *WebMD.com*. Last modified November 11, 2018. https://www.webmd.com/brain/mad-cow-disease-basics.

"Lazzaretto Vecchio." *AtlasObscura.com,* January 2, 2013. https://www.atlasobscura.com/places/lazzaretto-vecchio.

LePan, Nicholas. "Visualizing the History of Pandemics." *VisualCapitalist.com*, March 14, 2020. https://www.visualcapitalist.com/history-of-pandemics-deadliest.

Lepore, Jill. "What Our Contagion Fables Are Really About." *The New Yorker*, March 23, 2020. https://www.newyorker.com/magazine/2020/03/30/what-our-contagion-fables-are-really-about.

"Leprosy: Frequently Asked Questions." *Leprosy.org*. Last modified March 19, 2020. https://www.leprosy.org/leprosy-faqs.

"Leprosy: Symptoms, Treatments, History, and Causes." *WebMD.com*. Last modified April 23, 2019. https://www.webmd.com/skin-problems-and-treatments/guide/leprosy-symptoms-treatments-history.

Lipoff, Jules. "Eeek! The Actual Diseases That Inspired Vampires, Werewolves, and Zombies." *The Philadelphia Inquirer*, October 30, 2017. https://www.inquirer.com/philly/entertainment/movies /halloween-zombies-vampires-werewolves-disease-causes -20171030.html.

"List: These Famous People Have Coronavirus." *The Mercury News*. Last modified June 1, 2020. https://www.mercurynews.com/2020 /03/25/list-these-famous-people-have-coronavirus/.

Little, Becky. "When Mask-Wearing Rules in the 1918 Pandemic Faced Resistance." *History.com*, May 6, 2020. https://www.history.com /news/1918-spanish-flu-mask-wearing-resistance.

Li, Xiaojun, Elena E. Giorgi, Manukumar Honnayakanahalli Marichannegowda, Brian Foley, Chuan Xiao, Xiang-Peng Kong, Yue Chen et al. "Emergence of SARS-CoV-2 Through Recombination and Strong Purifying Selection." *Science Advances* 6, no. 27: (2020). https://advances.sciencemag.org/content/6/27/eabb9153.

Loughlin, Kevin. "Salk and Sabin: The Disease, the Rivalry and the Vaccine." *Hektoen International*. Last modified January 30, 2018. https://hekint.org/2018/01/30/salk-sabin-disease-rivalry-vaccine.

Luu, Christopher. "Tom Hanks and Rita Wilson Tested Positive for Coronavirus." *InStyle*, March 11, 2020. https://www.instyle.com /news/tom-hanks-rita-wilson-coronavirus.

Luy, Marc, Paola Di Giulio, Vanessa Di Lego, Patrick Lazarevič, and Markus Sauerberg. "Life Expectancy: Frequently Used, but Hardly Understood." *Gerontology* 66, no. 1 (2020): 95–104. https://www.karger.com/Article/Fulltext/500955.

"Lyme Disease." *CDC.gov*. Last modified December 16, 2019. https://www.cdc.gov/lyme/index.html.

Mahoney, Dennis, and Terence Chorba. "Romanticism, Mycobacterium, and the Myth of the Muse." *Emerging Infectious Diseases* 25, no. 3 (2019). https://wwwnc.cdc.gov/eid/article/25/3/ac-2503_article.

Maragakis, Lisa Lockerd. "Coronavirus Disease 2019 vs. the Flu." *HopkinsMedicine.org*. Last modified August 16, 2020. https://www .hopkinsmedicine.org/health/conditions-and-diseases/coronavirus /coronavirus-disease-2019-vs-the-flu.

Marineli, Filio, Gregory Tsoucalas, Marianna Karamanou, and George Androutsos. "Mary Mallon (1869–1938) and the History of Typhoid Fever." *Annals of Gastroenterology 26*, no. 2 (2013): 132–34. https://www.ncbi.nlm.nih.gov/pmc/articles/PMC3959940/.

Mark, Joshua J. "Thucydides on the Plague of Athens: Text and Commentary." *Ancient History Encyclopedia*. Last modified April 1, 2020. https://www.ancient.eu/article/1535/thucydides-on-the-plague-of-athens-text--commentar.

Marr, John S., and Charles H. Calisher. "Alexander the Great and West Nile Virus Encephalitis." *Emerging Infectious Diseases 9*, no. 12 (2003): 1599–1603. https://wwwnc.cdc.gov/eid/article/9/12/03-0288_article.

Mason, Matthew. "Microbiology: Tiniest Lifeforms Under the Microscope." *EnvironmentalScience.org*. Accessed August 3, 2020. https://www.environmentalscience.org/microbiology.

Matuschek, Christiane, Friedrich Moll, Heiner Fangerau, Johannes C. Fischer, Kurt Zänker, Martijn van Griensven, Marion Schneider et al. "The History and Value of Face Masks." *European Journal of Medical Research 25*, no. 23 (2020). https://www.ncbi.nlm.nih.gov/pmc/articles/PMC7309199.

McCue, Jack D. "The Contagious Patient." In *Clinical Methods: The History, Physical, and Laboratory Examinations*, ed. H. K. Walker, W. D. Hall, and J. W. Hurst. Boston: Butterworths, 1990.

McGraw, Elizabeth. "What Is a Super Spreader? An Infectious Disease Expert Explains." *TheConversation.com*. Last modified January 30, 2020. https://theconversation.com/what-is-a-super-spreader-an-infectious-disease-expert-explains-130756.

McMaken, Ryan. "Why States Don't Require Blood Tests for Marriages Anymore." *Mises.org*. Last modified January 30, 2018. https://mises.org/wire/why-states-dont-require-blood-tests-marriages-anymore.

McNeil Jr., Donald G. "Virus Deadly in Livestock Is No More, U.N. Declares." *The New York Times*, October 15, 2010. https://www.nytimes.com/2010/10/16/science/16pest.html.

_____. "New Ebola Vaccine Gives 100 Percent Protection." *The New York Times*, December 22, 2016. https://www.nytimes.com/2016/12/22/health/ebola-vaccine.html.

_____. "The Flu Vaccine Is Working Better Than Expected, C.D.C. Finds." *The New York Times*, February 16, 2018. https://www.nytimes.com/2018/02/15/health/flu-vaccine-effectiveness.html.

_____. "Why Don't We Have Vaccines Against Everything?" *The New York Times*, November 20, 2018. https://www.nytimes.com/2018/11/19/health/vaccines-poverty.html.

McVean, Ada. "Did You Know That Malaria Spawned the Gin and Tonic?" *McGill*, September 27, 2018. https://www.mcgill.ca/oss/article/did-you-know/malaria-reason-behind-gin-and-tonic.

Melzer, Emily. "Tuberculosis—A Romantic Disease?" *ThatsLifeScience.com*, November 13, 2017. http://thatslifesci.com/2017-11-13-a-romantic-disease-melzer.

"MERS-CoV Photos." *CDC.gov*. Last modified August 2, 2019. https://www.cdc.gov/coronavirus/mers/photos.html.

Merson, Michael H. "The HIV-AIDS Pandemic at 25—The Global Response." *New England Journal of Medicine*, no. 354 (2006): 2414–17. https://www.nejm.org/doi/full/10.1056/nejmp068074.

Meštrović, Tomislav, MD, PhD. "What Are Tropical Diseases?" *NewsMedical.com*. Last modified August 23, 2018. https://www.news-medical.net/health/What-are-Tropical-Diseases.aspx.

Mikkelson, David. "Fact Check: Is 'Ring Around the Rosie' About the Black Plague?" *Snopes.com*. Last modified November 17, 2000. https://www.snopes.com/fact-check/ring-around-rosie.

"Misconceptions About Seasonal Flu and Flu Vaccines." *CDC.gov*. Last modified September 1, 2020. https://www.cdc.gov/flu/prevent/misconceptions.htm.

"Mission, Role and Pledge." *CDC.gov*. Last modified May 13, 2019. https://www.cdc.gov/about/organization/mission.htm.

"MMR Vaccination." *CDC.gov*. Last modified March 28, 2019. https://www.cdc.gov/vaccines/vpd/mmr/public/index.html.

Mobilian, Julianne. "Scotts Miracle-Gro Shares Uptick of Gardening Statistics Related to Covid-19." *Garden Center Magazine*. Last modified June 8, 2020. https://www.gardencentermag.com/article/scotts-miracle-gro-shares-gardening-statistics-Covid-19.

Morrison, Jim. "A Virus Study You've Never Heard of Helped Us Understand Covid-19." *Smithsonian.com*, June 25, 2020. https://www.smithsonianmag.com/science-nature/virome-manhattan-jeffery-shaman-columbia-Covid-19-180975172/.

"Mycotoxins." *World Health Organization*. Last modified May 9, 2018. https://www.who.int/news-room/fact-sheets/detail/mycotoxins.

"Naming the Coronavirus Disease (Covid-19) and the Virus That Causes It." *World Health Organization*. Last modified August 16, 2020. https://www.who.int/emergencies/diseases/novel-coronavirus-2019/technical-guidance/naming-the-coronavirus-disease-(Covid-2019)-and-the-virus-that-causes-it.

"Necrotizing Fasciitis: Acting Fast Is Key." *CDC.gov*. Last modified December 31, 2019. https://www.cdc.gov/groupastrep/diseases-public/necrotizing-fasciitis.html.

"Neglected Tropical Diseases." *CDC.gov*. Last modified January 29, 2020. https://www.cdc.gov/globalhealth/ntd/index.html.

Newland, Christina. "The Prettiest Way to Die." *Literary Hub*, October 3, 2017. https://lithub.com/the-prettiest-way-to-die.

Ng, Philiana. "First Look: 'Chicago Fire,' 'Med' and 'PD' Team Up for Crossover Event." *Entertainment Tonight*, October 15, 2019. https://www.etonline.com/chicago-fire-med-and-pd-team-up-to-fight-flesh-eating-bacteria-in-crossover-sneak-peek-exclusive.

Ng, Ta-Chou, and Tzai-Hung Wen. "Spatially Adjusted Time-varying Reproductive Numbers: Understanding the Geographical Expansion of Urban Dengue Outbreaks." *Scientific Reports* 9, no. 19172 (2019). https://www.nature.com/articles/s41598-019-55574-0.pdf.

Nigam, P. K., and Anjana Nigam. "Botulinum Toxin." *Indian Journal of Dermatology* 55, no. 1 (2010): 8–14. https://www.ncbi.nlm.nih.gov/pmc/articles/PMC2856357.

Norkin, Leonard. "How the Human Immunodeficiency Deficiency Virus (HIV) Got Its Name." *NorkinVirology.com*, February 4, 2014. https://norkinvirology.wordpress.com/2014/02/04/how-the-human-immunodeficiency-deficiency-virus-hiv-got-its-name.

_____. "Jonas Salk and Albert Sabin: One of the Great Rivalries of Medical Science." *NorkinVirology.com*, May 14, 2014. https://norkinvirology.wordpress.com/2014/03/27/jonas-salk-and-albert-sabin-one-of-the-great-rivalries-of-medical-science.

_____. "Thucydides and the Plague of Athens." *NorkinVirology.com*, September 30, 2014. https://norkinvirology.wordpress.com/2014 /09/30/thucydides-and-the-plague-of-athens.

"Norovirus." *CDC.gov*. Last modified April 5, 2019. https://www.cdc .gov/norovirus/index.html.

Northern Arizona University. "Modern Lab Reaches Across the Ages to Resolve Plague DNA Debate." *Phys.org*. Last modified May 20, 2013. https://phys.org/news/2013-05-modern-lab-ages-plague -dna.html.

Noymer, Andrew, and Michel Garenne. "The 1918 Influenza Epidemic's Effects on Sex Differentials in Mortality in the United States." *Population and Development Review* 26, no. 3 (2000): 565–81. https://www.ncbi.nlm.nih.gov/pmc/articles/PMC2740912/.

O'Brien, Matt, and Sarah Rankin. "Virginia Rolls Out App to Alert Potential Covid-19 Exposure." *Time*, August 5, 2020. https://time .com/5876269/virginia-Covid19-exposure-alert-app/.

Ochab, Ewelina U. "What Does Gin and Tonic Have to Do with Malaria Prevention?" *Forbes*, April 26, 2018. https://www.forbes.com/sites /ewelinaochab/2018/04/26/what-does-gin-and-tonic-have-to-do -with-malaria-prevention/.

Oehler, Christina. "These 26 Celebrities Have Tested Positive for Coronavirus." *Health.com*, March 27, 2020. https://www.health.com /condition/infectious-diseases/coronavirus/celebrities-with -coronavirus.

"Official Mission Statements and Organizational Charts." *CDC.gov*. Last modified August 30, 2019. https://www.cdc.gov/about /organization/cio-orgcharts/index.html.

"Our History—Our Story." *CDC.gov*. Last modified December 4, 2018. https://www.cdc.gov/about/history/index.html.

"Outbreak: Ten of the Worst Pandemics in History." *MPHOnline.org*. Accessed July 29, 2020. https://www.mphonline.org/worst -pandemics-in-history.

"Outbreaks, Epidemics and Pandemics: What You Need to Know." *APIC.org*. Accessed July 20, 2020. https://apic.org/monthly_alerts /outbreaks-epidemics-and-pandemics-what-you-need-to-know.

"Pandemics That Changed History." *History.com*. Last updated April 1, 2020. https://www.history.com/topics/middle-ages/ pandemics-timeline.

Pappas, Stephanie. "Five Deadly Diseases Emerging from Global Warming." *LiveScience*, August 3, 2016. https://www.livescience .com/55632-deadly-diseases-emerge-from-global-warming.html.

Parker-Pope, Tara. "The Science of Chicken Soup." *The New York Times*, October 12, 2007. https://well.blogs.nytimes.com/2007/10/12 /the-science-of-chicken-soup/.

"Pathogen." *ScienceDaily*. Accessed July 9, 2020. https://www.sciencedaily.com/terms/pathogen.htm.

Pavia, Andrew T. "Germs on a Plane: Aircraft, International Travel, and the Global Spread of Disease." Oxford University Press, *The Journal of Infectious Diseases* 195, no. 5 (March 2007): 621–22. https://academic.oup.com/jid/article/195/5/621/841980.

"Personal Protective Equipment for Infection Control." *U.S. Food and Drug Administration*. FDA. Last modified February 10, 2020. https:// www.fda.gov/medical-devices/general-hospital-devices-and -supplies/personal-protective-equipment-infection-control.

Pietrangelo, Ann, and Rachel Nall. "Viral Gastroenteritis (Stomach Flu): Symptoms and Treatment." *Healthline*. Last modified March 7, 2019. https://www.healthline.com/health/viral-gastroenteritis.

"Plague." *CDC.gov*. Last modified July 23, 2020. https://www.cdc .gov/plague/index.html.

"Plague in the United States: Maps and Statistics." *CDC.gov*. Last modified November 25, 2019. https://www.cdc.gov/plague/maps /index.html.

"Plague." *World Health Organization*. Last modified April 26, 2012. https://www.who.int/ith/diseases/plague/en.

Porter, Katherine Anne. *Pale Horse, Pale Rider*. New York: Signet, 1936.

Preston, Richard. *The Hot Zone: The Terrifying True Story of the Origins of the Ebola Virus*. New York: Anchor Books, 1995.

"Preventing Illness Associated with Animal Contact ." *Minnesota Department of Health*. Last modified July 2013. https://www.health. state.mn.us/diseases/animal/animal.html.

"Prevention of Botulism." *CDC.gov*. Last modified June 7, 2019. https:// www.cdc.gov/botulism/prevention.html.

"Principles of Epidemiology." *CDC.gov*. Last modified May 18, 2012. https://www.cdc.gov/csels/dsepd/ss1978/lesson1/section11.html.

"Principles of Epidemiology: Lesson 6, Section 2|Self-Study Course SS1978|CDC." *CDC.gov*. Last modified September 15, 2016. https://www.cdc.gov/csels/dsepd/ss1978/lesson6/section2.html.

"Quarantine, Self-Isolation and Social Distancing for Covid-19." *Mayo Clinic*. Last modified August 6, 2020. https://www.mayoclinic.org/diseases-conditions/coronavirus/in-depth/coronavirus-quarantine-and-isolation/art-20484503.

"Rabies." *CDC.gov*. Last modified July 29, 2020. https://www.cdc.gov/rabies/index.html.

"Rabies." *World Health Organization*. Last modified August 12, 2020. https://www.who.int/news-room/fact-sheets/detail/rabies.

Rao, Tejal. "Food Supply Anxiety Brings Back Victory Gardens." *The New York Times*, March 25, 2020. https://www.nytimes.com/2020/03/25/dining/victory-gardens-coronavirus.html.

Razonable, Raymund R. "Antiviral Drugs for Viruses Other than Human Immunodeficiency Virus." *Mayo Clinic Proceedings* 86, no. 10 (2011): 1009–26. https://www.ncbi.nlm.nih.gov/pmc/articles/PMC3184032.

"Recommended Vaccines for Adults." *CDC.gov*. Last modified November 21, 2019. https://www.cdc.gov/vaccines/adults/rec-vac/index.html.

"Researchers Reconstruct 1918 Pandemic Influenza Virus; Effort Designed to Advance Preparedness." *ScienceDaily*, October 6, 2005. https://www.sciencedaily.com/releases/2005/10/051005230557.htm.

Rettner, Rachael. "Whooping Cough: Signs, Symptoms and Treatment." *LiveScience*, March 29, 2016. https://www.livescience.com/41956-whooping-cough-symptoms-treatment.html.

Riedel, Stefan. "Biological Warfare and Bioterrorism: A Historical Review." *Proceedings* 17, no. 4 (2004): 400–06. https://www.ncbi.nlm.nih.gov/pmc/articles/PMC1200679/.

Robbins, Jim. "How Forest Loss Is Leading to a Rise in Human Disease." *Yale Environment*, February 23, 2016. https://e360.yale.edu/features/how_forest_loss_is_leading_to_a_rise_in_human_disease_malaria_zika_climate_change.

Roland, James. "Quinine in Tonic Water: Is It Safe and What Are the Side Effects?" *Healthline*. Last modified September 18, 2018. https://www.healthline.com/health/quinine-in-tonic-water.

Roos, Dave. "How Crude Smallpox Inoculations Helped George Washington Win the War." *History.com*, May 13, 2020. https://www.history.com/news/smallpox-george-washington-revolutionary-war.

Rosen, William. *Justinian's Flea: Plague, Empire, and the Birth of Europe*. Philadelphia: Brécourt Academic, 2007.

Roser, Max, Sophie Ochmann, Hannah Behrens, Hannah Ritchie, and Bernadeta Dadonaite. "Eradication of Diseases." *OurWorldinData.org*, Last updated October 2018. https://ourworldindata.org/eradication-of-diseases.

_____, and Hannah Ritchie. "HIV/AIDS." *OurWorldinData.org*. Last updated November 2019. https://ourworldindata.org/hiv-aids.

"Rotavirus." *CDC.gov*. Last modified November 5, 2019. https://www.cdc.gov/rotavirus/index.html.

"Salmonella." *CDC.gov*. Last modified August 3, 2020. https://www.cdc.gov/salmonella/index.html.

Sartin, Jeffrey S. "Contagious Horror: Infectious Themes in Fiction and Film." *Clinical Medicine and Research* 17, no. 1 (2019): 41–46. Marshfield Clinic, June 2019. https://www.ncbi.nlm.nih.gov/pmc/articles/PMC6546279.

Schelden, Peter. "The Black Death: What Bubonic Plague Reveals About Covid-19 Coronavirus Pandemic." *MedicineNet.com*. Last modified March 19, 2020. https://www.medicinenet.com/script/main/art.asp?articlekey=229027.

Schmidt, Charles. "Coronavirus Researchers Tried to Warn Us." *The Atlantic*, June 13, 2020. https://www.theatlantic.com/health/archive/2020/06/scientists-predicted-coronavirus-pandemic/613003/.

Schwarcz, Joe. "A Spoonful of Sugar." *McGill*, January 20, 2017. https://www.mcgill.ca/oss/article/health-history/science-behind-spoonful-sugar.

Schwartzstein, Peter. "The History of Poisoning the Well." *Smithsonian.com*, February 13, 2019. https://www.smithsonianmag.com/history/history-well-poisoning-180971471.

Schweiker, William. "Plagues and the Pale Rider: Our Present Apocalypse." *The University of Chicago*, April 27, 2020. https://divinity.uchicago.edu/sightings/articles/plagues-and-pale-rider-our-present-apocalypse.

"The Science of the Ten Plagues." *LiveScience*, April 11, 2017. https://www.livescience.com/58638-science-of-the-10-plagues.html.

Scutti, Susan, and Katie Hunt. "Why Is the Plague Still a Thing in 2020? And Are You at Risk of Getting It?" *CNN*, August 19, 2020. https://www.cnn.com/2020/08/19/health/bubonic-plague-2020-california-wellness/index.html.

Seladi-Schulman, Jill. "Infections: Symptoms, Types, Causes, Treatments, List, and More." *Healthline*. Last modified November 5, 2018. https://www.healthline.com/health/infections.

"Selecting Viruses for the Seasonal Influenza Vaccine." *CDC.gov*. Last modified September 4, 2018. https://www.cdc.gov/flu/prevent/vaccine-selection.htm.

"Sexually Transmitted Diseases and Related Conditions." *CDC.gov*. Last modified November 4, 2016. https://www.cdc.gov/std/general/default.htm.

"Sexually Transmitted Infections (STIs)." *World Health Organization*. Last modified June 14, 2019. https://www.who.int/news-room/fact-sheets/detail/sexually-transmitted-infections-(stis).

Shanks, Daniel. "Pacific Island Societies Destabilised by Infectious Diseases. "*Journal of Military and Veterans' Health* 24, no.4 (October 2016). https://jmvh.org/article/pacific-island-societies-destabilised-by-infectious-diseases.

Shelley, Percy Bysshe. "Adonais: An Elegy on the Death of John Keats." *PoetryFoundation.org*. Accessed August 13, 2020. https://www.poetryfoundation.org/poems/45112/adonais-an-elegy-on-the-death-of-john-keats.

Shiel, William C. "Definition of Pestilence." *MedicineNet.com*. Last modified December 27, 2018. https://www.medicinenet.com/script/main/art.asp?articlekey=9101.

Shilts, Randy. *And the Band Played On: Politics, People, and the AIDS Epidemic*. New York: St. Martin's Press, 1987.

"Shingles." *CDC.gov*. Last modified August 14, 2019. https://www.cdc.gov/shingles/hcp/clinical-overview.html.

"Shiro Ishii." *PBS*. Accessed August 22, 2020. https://www.pbs.org/wgbh/americanexperience/features/weapon-biography-shiro-ishii.

Silver, Marc. "My Hand-Washing Song: Readers Offer Lyrics for a 20-Second Scrub." *NPR*. Last updated September 2020. https://www.npr.org/sections/goatsandsoda/2020/03/17/814221111/my-hand-washing-song-readers-offer-lyrics-for-a-20-second-scrub.

"Similarities and Differences Between Flu and Covid-19." *CDC.gov*. Last modified August 4, 2020. https://www.cdc.gov/flu/symptoms/flu-vs-Covid19.htm.

Sissons, Beth. "How to Treat a Cold or Flu at Home." *Medical News Today*, March 4, 2019. https://www.medicalnewstoday.com/articles/324607.

"Six Common Misconceptions about Immunization." *World Health Organization*. Last modified February 19, 2013. https://www.who.int/vaccine_safety/initiative/detection/immunization_misconceptions/en.

"Smallpox." *CDC.gov*. Last modified July 12, 2017. https://www.cdc.gov/smallpox/index.html.

"Smallpox." *National Institute of Allergy and Infectious Diseases*. Last modified May 15, 2020. https://www.niaid.nih.gov/diseases-conditions/smallpox.

Smith, Dale. "Will We Get a Coronavirus Vaccine in 2020? Everything You Need to Know." *CNET.com*. Last modified November 16, 2020. https://www.cnet.com/how-to/will-we-get-a-coronavirus-vaccine-in-2020-everything-you-need-to-know/.

Snowden, Frank M. *Epidemics and Society*. New Haven, CT: Yale University Press, 2020.

Sowards, Will. "You May Not Be Immune Forever—Why Boosters Are Important." *PassportHealth.com*, June 30, 2016. https://www.passporthealthusa.com/2016/06/why-boosters-are-important.

Steckelberg, James M. "Infection: Bacterial or Viral?" *Mayo Clinic*, September 7, 2017. https://www.mayoclinic.org/diseases-conditions/infectious-diseases/expert-answers/infectious-disease/faq-20058098.

Stein, Richard A. "Super-Spreaders in Infectious Diseases." *International Journal of Infectious Diseases* 15, no. 8 (2011): e510-e513. https://www.sciencedirect.com/science/article/pii/S1201971211000245.

Sterner, Carl S. "A Brief History of Miasmic Theory." *Carlsterner.com*, 2007. http://www.carlsterner.com/research/files/History_of _Miasmic_Theory_2007.pdf.

Strasser, Bruno J., and Thomas Schilich. "A History of the Medical Mask and the Rise of Throwaway Culture." *TheLancet.com*. Last modified May 22, 2020. https://www.thelancet.com/journals/lancet /article/PIIS0140-6736(20)31207-1/fulltext.

Stulberg, Brad. "Why We're All Gardening and Baking So Much." *OutsideOnline.org*, August 2, 2020. https://www.outsideonline .com/2415746/why-gardening-baking-popular-during-pandemic.

Summers, Bon. "The Deaths of the Brontë Family." *ILAB.gov*, December 30, 2009. https://ilab.org/articles/deaths-bronte-family.

Sun, Wei, and Amit K. Singh. "Plague Vaccine: Recent Progress and Prospects." *Nature Partner Journals* 4, no.11 (2019). https://www .nature.com/articles/s41541-019-0105-9.

"Testing for Covid-19." *CDC.gov*. Last modified August 16, 2020. https://www.cdc.gov/coronavirus/2019-ncov/symptoms-testing /testing.html.

"Tetanus." *CDC.gov*. Last modified February 28, 2019. https://www .cdc.gov/tetanus/about/prevention.html.

"Tetanus." *World Health Organization*. Last modified July 16, 2020. https://www.who.int/news-room/fact-sheets/detail/tetanus.

Than, Ker. "Massive Population Drop Found for Native Americans, DNA Shows." *National Geographic*, December 5, 2011. https://www.nationalgeographic.com/news/2011/12/111205-native -americans-europeans-population-dna-genetics-science.

Thavaselvam, Duraipandian, and Rajagopalan Vijayaraghavan. "Biological Warfare Agents." *Journal of Pharmacy and Bioallied Sciences* 2, no. 3 (2010): 179–88. https://www.ncbi.nlm.nih.gov/pmc /articles/PMC3148622.

Thomas, Jen. "Facts and Statistics About the Flu." *Healthline*. Last modified November 19, 2018. https://www.healthline.com/health /influenza/facts-and-statistics.

Thompson, Stuart A. "How Long Will a Vaccine Really Take?" *The New York Times*, April 30, 2020. https://www.nytimes.com /interactive/2020/04/30/opinion/coronavirus-Covid-vaccine.html.

"A Timeline of HIV and AIDS." *HIV.gov.* Accessed August 3, 2020. https://www.hiv.gov/hiv-basics/overview/history/hiv-and-aids -timeline.

"The Top Ten Causes of Death." *World Health Organization.* Last modified May 24, 2018. https://www.who.int/news-room/fact -sheets/detail/the-top-10-causes-of-death.

"Top Twenty Questions About Vaccination." *HistoryofVaccines.org.* Accessed July 30, 2020. https://www.historyofvaccines.org/index .php/content/articles/top-20-questions-about-vaccination.

Torrey, Trisha. "Phases of a Pandemic." *Verywell Health.* Last modified September 21, 2020. https://www.verywellhealth.com /understanding-a-pandemic-2615488.

"Tropical Diseases." *World Health Organization.* Last modified August 18, 2015. https://www.who.int/topics/tropical_diseases/en.

Trueba, Gabriel, and Micah Dunthorn. "Many Neglected Tropical Diseases May Have Originated in the Paleolithic or Before: New Insights from Genetics." *Public Library of Science Neglected Tropical Diseases* 6, no. 3, (2012): 1393. https://www.ncbi.nlm.nih.gov/pmc /articles/PMC3313944.

"Tuberculosis." *CDC.gov.* Last modified December 12, 2016. https://www.cdc.gov/tb/worldtbday/history.htm.

"Tuberculosis on Aircraft." In *Tuberculosis and Air Travel: Guidelines for Prevention and Control,* Geneva: U.S. National Library of Medicine, January 1, 1970.

"Types of Influenza Viruses." *CDC.gov.* Last modified November 18, 2019. https://www.cdc.gov/flu/about/viruses/types.htm.

Uhllmann, Agnes. "Pasteur-Koch: Distinctive Ways of Thinking About Infectious Disease." *Microbe* 2, no. 8 (2007): 383–87. http:// www.antimicrobe.org/h04c.files/history/Microbe%202007%20 Pasteur-Koch.pdf.

"The U.S. Government and the World Health Organization." *KFF.org.* Last modified April 16, 2020. https://www.kff.org/global-health -policy/fact-sheet/the-u-s-government-and-the-world-health -organization.

"Vaccine Development, Testing, and Regulation." *HistoryofVaccines. com.* Accessed July 12, 2020. https://www.historyofvaccines.org /content/articles/vaccine-development-testing-and-regulation.

"Vaccines: What Would Happen If We Stopped Vaccinations." *CDC. gov*. Last modified June 29, 2018. https://www.cdc.gov/vaccines /vac-gen/whatifstop.htm.

"Vaccine Testing and Approval Process." *CDC.gov*. Last modified May 1, 2014. https://www.cdc.gov/vaccines/basics/test-approve.html.

"Vaccine Timeline." *Immunize.org*. Last modified July 24, 2020. https://www.immunize.org/timeline/.

"Vampire History." *History.com*. Last updated February 21, 2020. https://www.history.com/topics/folklore/vampire-history.

"Vector-Borne Diseases." *World Health Organization*. Last modified August 10, 2020. https://www.who.int/news-room/fact-sheets /detail/vector-borne-diseases.

"Viral Gastroenteritis (Stomach Flu)." *Mayo Clinic*. Last modified October 16, 2018. https://www.mayoclinic.org/diseases-conditions /viral-gastroenteritis/symptoms-causes/syc-20378847.

"Wash Your Lyrics." *WashYourLyrics.com*. Accessed August 11, 2020. https://washyourlyrics.com/.

Waxman, Olivia B. "Did the Ten Plagues of Egypt Really Happen?" *Time*, March 2, 2020. https://time.com/5561441/passover-10 -plagues-real-history/.

Wells, Diana. "Zoonosis: Definition, Types, and Diseases List." *Healthline*. Last modified July 20, 2017. https://www.healthline.com /health/zoonosis.

Wenzl, Roy. "How Diseases Spread: Ways People Have Tried to Explain Pandemics Through History." *History.com*, April 8, 2020. https://www.history.com/news/how-infectious-diseases-spread -myth-superstition-theories.

Wessel, Lindzi. "Feed a Cold, Starve a Fever? Here's What Science Says." *STATNews.com*, September 8, 2016. https://www.statnews .com/2016/09/08/feed-cold-starve-fever-science/.

"West Nile Virus." *CDC.gov*. Last modified June 3, 2020. https://www.cdc.gov/westnile/index.html.

"What Are Antibiotics and How Do They Work?" *Microbiology Society*. Last modified August 12, 2020. https://microbiologysociety.org /members-outreach-resources/outreach-resources/antibiotics -unearthed/antibiotics-and-antibiotic-resistance/what-are -antibiotics-and-how-do-they-work.html.

"What Are HIV and AIDS?" *HIV.gov*. Last modified June 18, 2020. https://www.hiv.gov/hiv-basics/overview/about-hiv-and-aids/what-are-hiv-and-aids.

"What Can You Catch in Restrooms?" *WebMD*. Last modified August 2, 2020. https://www.webmd.com/balance/features/what-can-you-catch-in-restrooms.

"What Is Botulinum Toxin Used For?" *MedicineNet.com*. Last modified July 20, 2020. https://www.medicinenet.com/what_is_botulinum_toxin_used_for/article.htm.

"What Is Ebola Virus Disease?" *CDC.gov*. Last modified November 5, 2019. https://www.cdc.gov/vhf/ebola/about.html.

"What Is Rabies?" *World Health Organization*. Last modified September 25, 2018. https://www.who.int/rabies/about/en.

"What's the Difference Between a Pandemic, an Epidemic, Endemic, and an Outbreak?" *IntermountainHealthcare.org*, April 2, 2020. https://intermountainhealthcare.org/blogs/topics/live-well/2020/04/whats-the-difference-between-a-pandemic-an-epidemic-endemic-and-an-outbreak/.

"What You Should Know About Flu Antiviral Drugs." *CDC.gov*. Last modified April 22, 2019. https://www.cdc.gov/flu/treatment/whatyoushould.htm.

"Where Did HIV Come From?" *TheAidsInstitue.org*. Accessed August 1, 2020. https://www.theaidsinstitute.org/education/aids-101/where-did-hiv-come-0.

"Where Is Your Dog Coming From?" *CDC.gov*. Last modified December 18, 2018. https://www.cdc.gov/importation/bringing-an-animal-into-the-united-states/dog-origin.html.

"WHO Best Practices for Naming of New Human Infectious Diseases." *World Health Organization*. Last modified May 15, 2015. https://www.who.int/topics/infectious_diseases/naming-new-diseases/en.

"WHO Campaigns." *World Health Organization*. Last modified August 9, 2020. https://www.who.int/campaigns.

"WHO Pandemic Phase Descriptions and Main Actions by Phase." *World Health Organization*. Last modified July 2, 2020. https://www.who.int/influenza/resources/documents/pandemic_phase_descriptions_and_actions.pdf.

"The WHO Pandemic Phases." In *Pandemic Influenza Preparedness and Response: A WHO Guidance Document*. Geneva: World Health Organization, July 2020.

"Why Are We Involved." *CDC.gov*. Last modified October 24, 2019. https://www.cdc.gov/polio/why-are-we-involved/index.htm.

Wilford, John Noble. "Malaria Is a Likely Killer in King Tut's Post-Mortem." *The New York Times*, February 16, 2010. https://www.nytimes.com/2010/02/17/science/17tut.html.

Wong, Kate. "Navy Recruits Wash Their Hands of Coughs and Colds." *Scientific American*, August 1, 2001. https://www.scientificamerican.com/article/navy-recruits-wash-their.

Ye, Zi-Wei, and Shuofeng Yuan. "Zoonotic Origins of Human Coronaviruses." *International Journal of Biological Sciences* 16, no. 10 (2020):1686–1697. https://www.ncbi.nlm.nih.gov/pmc/articles/PMC7098031.

"Yellow Fever." *CDC.gov*. Last modified January 15, 2019. https://www.cdc.gov/yellowfever/index.html.

"Yellow Fever." *MayoClinic.org*. Last modified September 7, 2018. https://www.mayoclinic.org/diseases-conditions/yellow-fever/symptoms-causes/syc-20353045.

Yuill, Bessie. "Typhoid Mary Was a Real, Asymptomatic Carrier Who Caused Multiple Outbreaks." *Discover Magazine*, July 2, 2020. https://www.discovermagazine.com/health/typhoid-mary-was-a-real-asymptomatic-carrier-who-caused-multiple-outbreaks.

"Zombie Preparedness." *Centers for Disease Control and Prevention*. Last modified October 11, 2018. https://www.cdc.gov/cpr/zombie/index.htm.

"Zoonotic Diseases." *Centers for Disease Control and Prevention*. Last modified July 14, 2017. https://www.cdc.gov/onehealth/basics/zoonotic-diseases.html.

ACKNOWLEDGMENTS

Writing *The Big Book of Infectious Disease Trivia* was an immersive, surreal experience. I was quarantined with my own family due to the COVID-19 pandemic and found it surprisingly comforting to research the effects that infectious diseases and deadly pandemics have had on the world. I have never felt more connected to history and the generations that have come before, although I admit I'm more aware than ever of my own mortality.

Many thanks to everyone at Ulysses Press for helping me bring this book to life, especially Claire Sielaff, who gave me a fascinating project to work on right when I needed it most, and Tyanni Niles, who guided the book from draft to completion. Sending a book into the world is a group effort, and I could not have done it without a supportive editorial team.

Special thanks also go to my friend Eli Gorman, who answered my questions about infectious diseases and was always generous with her knowledge of public health. And if my book had a patron saint, it would be Anthony Fauci, MD, a modern-day hero who has been a font of knowledge and soft-spoken wisdom in a very peculiar year.

And big, big love to my incredible husband, Jay, and our sons, Patrick and Lucas. The Marvel Cinematic Universe, Friday night pizza, garden conversations, Starbucks runs, and Pokémon raids have kept me going this past year.

Thanks for putting up with me when I quoted disease statistics or freaked out about the state of the world. You give me a reason to believe that it really will get better, and I'm so glad I get to go through life with you guys on my side!

And lastly, many thanks to you, dear reader, for being as curious about infectious diseases as I am. Happy reading, and don't forget to wash your hands!

ABOUT THE AUTHOR

Kristina Wright is a writer and an editor who lives in Virginia with her husband, two sons, two dogs, one cat, and one parrot. She holds a BA in English from Charleston Southern University and an MA in humanities from Old Dominion University, and she has taught composition and world mythology at the college level. Her essays and articles have appeared in a variety of publications, including the *Washington Post*, *USA Today*, and the *Huffington Post*, and she is the digital editor at *Your Teen for Parents* magazine.

Kristina has also written novels for Harlequin and HarperCollins and has edited more than a dozen fiction anthologies for Cleis Press. She shares her passion for books and entertainment at BookBub and writes a monthly book review column at the *Washington Independent Review of Books*. Kristina is an enthusiastic coffee drinker who loves baking bread, researching obscure history, reading thrillers, watching reruns of *Friends* and *Grey's Anatomy*, and planning family trips where everyone has fun and no one complains. When the COVID-19 pandemic is over and she can travel again, Kristina plans to go to Italy—alone.